Praise for
Living Well with Pain and Illness

"The cultivation of mindfulness can make a profound difference in how we relate to pain and whether chronic pain conditions need to turn into endless suffering and misery. This has been known over the past 2,600 years and is now being supported by studies in both medicine and neuroscience. In this book, Vidyamala makes the practice of befriending your experience through mindfulness, however unpleasant or pleasant it may be, both commonsensical and compelling. I admire her tremendously. This is a beautiful and very important book. It could save your life — and give it back to you."

JON KABAT-ZINN, PHD, AUTHOR OF *FULL CATASTROPHE LIVING*
AND *COMING TO OUR SENSES*

"This is a wonderful work, one of those books where you know within a few pages that it is going to be worth stopping everything else in order to make time to read it. The book is a moving and compelling invitation to bring a radically new way of working with the fact of our pain. It is a book of enormous tenderness and honesty. Here is wise guidance on how we can move beyond our natural resistance to our pain to a willingness to be with it, and how we can live with greater ease by turning toward what we most fear about our pain and suffering."

MARK WILLIAMS, COAUTHOR OF *MINDFULNESS-BASED COGNITIVE THERAPY FOR
DEPRESSION* AND *THE MINDFUL WAY THROUGH DEPRESSION* AND PROFESSOR
OF CLINICAL PSYCHOLOGY AND WELLCOME PRINCIPAL RESEARCH FELLOW,
DEPARTMENT OF PSYCHIATRY, UNIVERSITY OF OXFORD, UK

"Vidyamala Burch has practiced mindfulness for many years, and she has applied the practice to the relief of physical suffering. She has now embodied the fruits of her extensive experience in a very readable and useful book. I hope that *Living Well with Pain and Illness* will have a wide circulation in a world where, despite all our progress, there is still so much suffering, some of it unnecessary."

URGYEN SANGHARAKSHITA

"It is one thing to have our pain and emotions and another to be ruled by them, one thing to live our life and another to live in our thoughts about our life, one thing to make choices according to what we hold as important and another to helplessly act as our habits will have us do. This wonderful book helps us to appreciate these differences. The act of reading it alone may bring a small measure of space, life, freedom, warmth, and gentleness to your life. Following the direction it suggests could bring you much more and radically change your life for the better."

LANCE M. MCCRACKEN, PHD, CLINICAL PSYCHOLOGIST AND CLINICAL LEAD, BATH CENTER FOR PAIN SERVICES, ROYAL NATIONAL HOSPITAL FOR RHEUMATIC DISEASES AND CENTER OF PAIN RESEARCH, SCHOOL FOR HEALTH, UNIVERSITY OF BATH

"This is an excellent self-help book for sufferers of chronic illnesses. It guides the reader in how to deal with pain, illness, frustrations, anxieties, and even life itself. Vidyamala has written a beautiful, profound, yet easy to understand book on how to live happily, regardless of what state of pain or difficulty you are in. A definite must-read for my patients, students, and colleagues in health care. A milestone book on living mindfulness fully."

TONY FERNANDO, MD, PSYCHIATRIST, UNIVERSITY OF AUCKLAND, FACULTY OF MEDICAL AND HEALTH SCIENCES, NEW ZEALAND

"In describing her own journey with pain, Vidyamala has written a definitive guide to the practice of meditation with pain and illness. She explains how we have a choice as to whether or not we suffer with pain, and she teaches us a quiet and reflective attitude of acceptance and kindness toward ourselves and others. Vidyamala describes how, through becoming more aware of our body and its sensations, the pain diminishes. I am happy to recommend this useful book to the members of my support group."

"This book, while acknowledging the complexity of living with pain and illness, suggests creative ways to live with these challenges. Vidyamala draws not only from her own experience with chronic pain but also from the experiences of her many students who have learned, through Breathworks, to live with their pain more skillfully using mindfulness. She demonstrates skills and understanding that can help us all move through life with greater ease whatever our 'particular version of the human predicament' may be."

"Vidyamala has made an insightful contribution to the current dialogue between mindfulness and the fields of medicine and psychology. Rooted in her own experience, this book will be a great support both to those living with pain and those endeavoring to find new ways of working with pain and illness."

LIVING WELL
WITH PAIN & ILLNESS

The Mindful Way

to Free Yourself

from Suffering

VIDYAMALA BURCH

LIVING WELL
WITH PAIN & ILLNESS

SOUNDS TRUE
BOULDER, COLORADO

Sounds True, Inc. Boulder, CO 80306

© 2010 Vidyamala Burch
Foreword © 2008 Amanda C. de C. Williams

Published 2010.

First published in the United Kingdom by Piatkus, an imprint of Little, Brown
Book Group.

ISBN 978-1-59179-747-0

Cover design by Lisa Kerans
Book design by Karen Polaski
Printed in the U.S.A.

NOTE
All the techniques and methods introduced in this book can be used alongside
medical treatment. They are not intended as a substitute, and anyone with
undiagnosed pain or any other symptoms they are concerned about should seek
advice from a qualified medical practitioner or suitable therapist.

Grateful acknowledgment is made to reproduce the following:

Page 49, from *Rumi: Selected Poems*, translated by Coleman Barks, © 1995. Permission granted by Coleman Barks.

Page 65, "Ah, Not to Be Cut Off" from *Ahead of All the Parting* by Rainer Maria Rilke, translated by Stephen Mitchell, © 1995 by Stephen Mitchell. Permission granted by Modern Library, a division of Random House.

Page 67, from *Full Catastrophe Living* by Jon Kabat-Zinn, © 2004. Permission granted by Little, Brown, London.

Page 70–72, from *Waking* by Matthew Sanford, © 2006 by Matthew Sanford. Permission granted by Rodale, Inc.

Page 73, "Wild Geese" from *Dream Work* by Mary Oliver, © 1986 by Mary Oliver. Permission granted by Grove/Atlantic, Inc.

Page 77, from *Heartwood: Meditations on Southern Oaks* by Rumi and William Guion, translated by Coleman Barks, © 1998. Permission granted by Coleman Barks.

Page 86, from *Trust in Mind: The Rebellion of Chinese Zen* © Mu Soeng, 2004. Permission granted by Wisdom Publications, Somerville, Massachusetts. wisdompubs.org

Page 93, from *Rumi: Selected Poems*, translated by Coleman Barks, © 1995. Permission granted by Coleman Barks.

Page 123, from *Great Fool*, by Ryokan, University of Hawai'i Press, 1996.

Page 131, from *Where Many Rivers Meet* by David Whyte, © 1990. Permission granted by Many Rivers Press, Langley, Washington. davidwhyte.com

Page 145 and epigraph, from *Rumi: Hidden Music*, translated by Maryam Mafi and Azima Melita Kolin, © 2001 by Azima Melita and Maryam Mafi. Permission granted by HarperCollins Publishers Ltd.

Page 165, from *Rilke's Book of Hours: Love Poems to God* by Rainer Maria Rilke, translated by Anita Barrows and Joanna Macy, © 1996 by Anita Barrows and Joanna Macy. Permission granted by Riverhead Books, an imprint of Penguin Group (USA) Inc.

Page 224, "Autobiography in Five Short Chapters" from *There's a Hole in My Sidewalk*, by Portia Nelson, © by Portia Nelson. Beyond Words Publishing, Hillsboro, Oregon.

Pages 232–233, "Pleasant and Unpleasant Events Diary" adapted from "Awareness of Pleasant or Unpleasant Events Calendar" from *Full Catastrophe Living* by Jon Kabat-Zinn, Little Brown, London, 2004.

＊

For all people with difficulties everywhere.
May this book give you some peace and ease.
For Sona, Ratnaguna, and the Breathworks community, with deep
gratitude for sharing my vision and making it real.

*

Do not look back, my friend
No one knows how the world ever began.
Do not fear the future, nothing lasts forever.
If you dwell on the past or the future
You will miss the moment.

RUMI, *HIDDEN MUSIC*, TRANSLATED BY
MARYAM MAFI AND AZIMA MALITA KOLIN

Contents

PART VI: MINDFULNESS AT ALL TIMES

Foreword

P ain is such a universal experience, and yet, for all its familiarity, there is a vast amount about it that we don't understand and for which we barely have adequate concepts. I have worked in the field of pain (mainly in group treatment using cognitive behavioral methods) for over twenty years and have contributed to the research literature on the effectiveness of cognitive behavioral methods. I have learned a tremendous amount from several thousand patients treated at INPUT Pain Management Unit at St. Thomas's Hospital in London, where I directed research activities, and from studying the research literature and evidence. But being introduced to Vidyamala and her work, as she describes it in this book, has added a new dimension to my thinking about the psychology of pain.

Most of the difficulties in conceptualizing pain arise from the profound dualism of Western thinking, in which an autonomous spirit floats free, observing and organizing the body in which it officially resides. This way of thinking spreads confusion and undermines an integrated understanding of ourselves. By drawing on non-Western philosophies, we may find more effective ways to represent, inevitably in a simplified way, the extraordinarily complex and recursive processes underlying the experiences of pain. *Living Well with Pain and Illness* takes such ideas, and some of the practices and stances that accompany them, and applies them to the problems of living with pain in a way that is deeply inspirational, and at the same time, completely practical. The spirit of scientific curiosity, of accountability, of honesty, and of wanting to build on the best of current understanding, is exemplified in this book. This spirit distinguishes the philosophy and practice of mindfulness and meditative methods as applied to pain from many of the alternative and complementary treatment methods with which it is sometimes grouped.

Pain arises from a warning system that is superbly efficient; it is immediate, and it demands our attention. Even so, it is not only driven by warnings of external dangers. What we experience as pain is a balance between, on the one hand, signals of what is happening outside and inside our bodies and, on the other, what our brains judge to be priorities and worth our attention. As with any complex system, this balance can get disrupted, generating false alarms, amplifying pain, overestimating threat, diverting attention to a pain that is already too familiar. The pain is absolutely real, but there is some room to maneuver around or to disengage from the threat, the distress, and the insistence of the pain experience. This maneuvering can be summarized as changing the relationship with pain.

I met Vidyamala in 2004, several years after she had written to me asking about how to best evaluate her work with Breathworks, and hoping to share insights in pain management. Hers seems to be a model approach: it is not enough to convince yourself that your approach is working; you need evidence as well. Her work was driven by patients and her own scientific curiosity, and her description of that work was expressed with passion, as was her wish to be account-able for the quality of the work, both to patients and to the wider pain-treatment field.

Evidence is accumulating for the efficacy of this way of managing pain. One of the earliest studies on mindfulness, by Jon Kabat-Zinn and his group,[1] involved people with chronic/persistent pain, but it was several decades later that the research literature started to develop, notably with studies from the Bath Pain Management Center.[2] From the start, Vidyamala and her colleagues have taken a thoughtful stance toward evaluating their group work, and particularly toward trying to understand the processes by which mindfulness changes the experience of pain and its impact on the person with pain. She reminds us that the term "rehabilitation" means "re-inhabiting," and all the methods in this book help the person with pain to re-inhabit his or her body with greater harmony and ease, no matter how painful the body may feel, rather than trying to fight it or block out its messages.

People with pain, who are too often characterized in the medical literature in terms of inactivity, avoidance, caution, and withdrawal from everyday life, often describe their experience in terms of "fighting the pain" or "trying not to give in to the pain." However, they can never "win" outright, and so they most often feel as if life is a permanent battlefield. This book describes instead how to negotiate peace with pain, to understand and find common ground—even, one might say, to plant flowers there. There are not only helpful descriptions and discussions of meditation and related practices in the context of persistent pain, but also an honest account of overcoming resistance and perverse attitudes, and thoughtful sections about physical positions that take account of pain. Vidyamala fully acknowledges the difficulties of pain rather than telling a tale of false comfort. She wrote the book in paced spells at the computer, because the time she can sit is limited by the buildup of pain, demonstrating acceptance and kindliness. Her struggles are described with humor, affection, and understanding, and it is clear that she truly listens to the struggles of other people.

This is one of the most generous and empathic books I have read. Nobody with an open mind could fail to learn from it. Readers with and without pain will recognize eloquent descriptions of the traps we fall into when we struggle to avoid what we don't want in our lives. Vidyamala brings an intuitive voice to a thoughtful, thorough, but not uncritical description of mindfulness and meditation theory and practice. She uses her own experiences, particularly her experience of her own pain, but without a trace of self-absorption or solipsism. The way she describes living with pain is anything but separate and mystical: it is very alive, connected, aware of the self and of others. I remember particularly how this came across at a packed workshop at the British Pain Society meeting in 2006. Vidyamala and her colleagues Gary and Sona held the complete attention of doctors, physiotherapists, psychologists, nurses, and others as they described their work, answered questions, and took the audience through some mindfulness exercises.

When she first contacted me in 2001, Vidyamala wrote: "I do love this work and am often very moved and inspired by the people I meet," and that was exactly what emerged from talking to her — a completely authentic desire to share, a capacity to integrate the details of people's struggles with pain with the larger picture of pain and the various dimensions in which help was constructed, and a drive to provide the highest possible standard of help that she and her colleagues could manage. The work of Vidyamala and her close colleagues comes from not only their beliefs, but from a deep emotional commitment to easing the suffering of anyone who lives with pain of any sort. This book comes from the same spirit.

DR. AMANDA C. DE C. WILLIAMS
READER IN CLINICAL HEALTH PSYCHOLOGY
UNIVERSITY COLLEGE, LONDON

Acknowledgments

Many people have contributed to this book. It certainly could never have been written without them. Thanks especially to Vishvapani, who worked on the text with me and brought dedication, fine intelligence, and a pursuit of excellence to his work as my editor, as well as a shared love of the topic. Helen Stanton at Piatkus has also been an encouraging presence throughout the writing of the original UK edition, and her experience and clear eye have helped us make the book the best we could. Geoffrey Moorhouse and Marilyn and Michael Dugdale were encouraging and helpful in the early stages when I was trying to get a publisher and they helped ensure the success of this quest. Thanks also to Caro Edwards and Bodhaniya, who made generous financial donations to the project, and to Subhuti and Mokshapriya, whose Welsh cottages gave me periods of concentrated work free from the distractions of life at home. The team at Sounds True in the United States has been wonderful in being enthusiastic about this book and preparing it for re-release to the American market. Haven Iverson has been particularly helpful and always passionate and considerate.

The UK's Millennium Commission gives grants for disabled people who want to contribute to the community, and it helped me start the Peace of Mind project in 2001. Without this initial investment I doubt that Breathworks, as the project was later called, would have begun. My deep thanks go to the cofounders of Breathworks, Sona Fricker and Gary Hennessey (Ratnaguna). They share my aspiration to make mindfulness available for people who are suffering from pain, illness, or stress, and much of the content of this book has been developed by the three of us.

Padmadarshini (Rosey Cole) was instrumental in developing the mindful movement program. She is a gifted yoga teacher who has been consistently generous with her time and talents. I am also indebted to Donna Farhi for her in-depth exploration of the breath, especially in *The Breathing Book*. This helped me develop the thinking behind chapter 7. Pete Moore of the Persistent Pain Program in the United Kingdom provided inspiration for part 6.

Dr. Amanda Williams has been tremendously supportive of my work and has helped me find ways to engage with the scientific and medical world of chronic pain. I have the greatest respect for her unwavering commitment to responding to the human aspect of pain and suffering, regardless of the cause.

Dr. Jon Kabat-Zinn has also been generous with his time and support. I first came across his work when I was still struggling to establish an effective meditation practice while living with a painful body. His approach was like an oasis in a desert.

I feel deep gratitude to Sangharakshita, my Buddhist teacher, who has translated Buddhist teachings into a form accessible to a modern Western woman like myself. Quite simply, his teachings have changed my life. In founding the Western Buddhist Order he established a community within which I am supported to follow the Buddhist path.

Thanks also to my friends, family, and personal assistants, who have been so patient as I've immersed myself in writing, allowing me the space to get on with it. I am especially grateful to my partner, Sona, who has been a source of kindness and stability. Thanks also to my parents, who helped me with so much kindness and generosity to come to terms with my disability as best I could. They have always exemplified the enterprising, pioneering spirit of New Zealanders and encouraged these qualities in me.

Finally, I thank all the people who are ill and living with pain who have involved themselves in Breathworks over the years. Their courage and openness have helped me formulate the material in this book. Many have also generously shared their stories, which are included in the book, and I've changed their names to protect their privacy.

Introduction:
Using This Book

※

In a small independent bookshop in London in 1990, I picked
up a book called *Who Dies?*[1] It included exercises to help people
approach illness and death with dignified awareness by turning
toward their experience, and one chapter dealt specifically with ways
to work with physical pain. I read it avidly. Already I had lived with
constant pain for fourteen years following a spinal injury, and as I
read, I felt tremendous relief. For the first time I'd found an approach
to living with pain that I intuitively knew to be true.

Although I'd already been meditating for several years, this was the
first time that I'd come across explicit guidance in how to meditate
with physical pain. What was so radical and compelling was the
message of opening to the pain in a kindly and accepting way rather
than continually trying to defeat and overcome it. I embraced this
message and began to apply it to my situation, for I knew my deeply
entrenched habit of battling my pain simply caused more pain — and
I wanted that fight to end.

This book is dedicated to anyone who finds him- or herself in the
situation of that embattled young woman and who wants new ways
to live with pain and illness or other long-term difficulties, regardless
of their cause. I've written it in the hope that it will help you in the
way that I was helped by *Who Dies?* and other books — as well as by
the teachers with whom I've had the good fortune to study during my
twenty years of mindfulness practice. Mindfulness is a special kind of
awareness that is attentive and warmly engaged with each moment

of life, and for me, it has been a lifesaver. It has shown me how I can be creative with my mental and emotional states rather than reactive. This has helped me to lay down my weapons and come to terms with my situation with maturity and peace. I still have pain, but the pain of fighting that pain has eased, and my quality of life has improved beyond recognition.

In 2004 I cofounded Breathworks, a nonprofit organization that offers mindfulness-based strategies to others living with pain, illness, and stress. We teach the methods introduced in this book, usually to groups of ten to fifteen people who meet for eight weekly sessions. The people I meet always inspire me. When human beings confront real difficulty and have no option but to dig deep within, inner nobility often comes forth. I continually learn lessons myself as I watch people inch their way, week by week, back to a life that feels worth living.

Over the years of running Breathworks, I'm often asked for materials by people unable to attend a course that would enable them to benefit from the magic of mindfulness. This book is in part a response to those requests, and I hope you will find it interesting and practically useful. I've also written it with a strong sense of how I myself felt all those years ago when I first faced the loneliness of disability and chronic pain with few skills to help me. Over subsequent years I have made many mistakes, but I have also learned many valuable lessons, and if this book can help even a few people find an easier way through their own journey with pain and illness, then I will feel it has been well worth writing.

HOW TO USE THIS BOOK

The book is divided into sections covering the underlying principles of a mindful approach to living with pain and illness, as well as practical guidance and exercises.

Principles

- Part 1 starts with my own story of living with pain. It looks at the nature of pain and describes how we can find a new relationship with it using mindfulness.
- Part 2 explores mindfulness and how it can bring wholeness, even if your body is injured or ill.

Practical Guidance

- Part 3 shows you how to come home to your body through breath awareness and mindful movement.
- Part 4 explores meditation in more detail and offers useful tips.
- Part 5 introduces three formal meditation practices.
- Part 6 looks at how you can take mindfulness into your daily life.

From my own experience, I've learned the importance of applying mindfulness to the whole of my life. The benefits will be lessened if you meditate but lose awareness during the day or don't bring mindfulness to how you move your body or are habitually gripped by destructive habits of thinking and speaking. So the mindfulness program introduced here covers all aspects of your life: breath and body awareness, mindful movement, transforming your mind and emotions with meditation, and bringing mindfulness to your daily life. No one practices mindfulness perfectly, but if you bring mindfulness to all the moments of the day, no matter how imperfect each moment may be, this will open the door to a dramatically improved life.

The main focus of the book is physical pain, but the mindfulness techniques are relevant to illness of any sort. They will help you manage your energy and fatigue and improve your quality of life. The techniques are also relevant to mental and emotional suffering, such as stress, anxiety, and depression.

Living with pain myself, I know how off-putting it is to be confronted by a long, densely written, and heavy book. With that in mind I have written this in a convenient format and divided the book into short sections, so you can dip in and out of it at your own pace. You may want to start with the exploration of the breath and movement in part 3, or perhaps the meditation practices in part 5, but the other chapters will help you understand more fully what you're doing.

Making mindfulness an integral part of your life takes practice. Appendix 1 includes a weekly guide outlining how you can systematically learn the various practices in this book. This will help you get the most from the program and develop a satisfying and sustainable schedule of learning over several weeks.

It also helps to be guided in these practices. I recommend that alongside the book you use the "led" meditations that I've recorded, and these are available via the Sounds True website: soundstrue.com/burch. Listening to these exercises will bring to life the relevant aspect of mindfulness in a more vivid and meaningful way than simply reading about it, so I strongly encourage you to make time to listen to these tracks. You will also gain the most benefit from mindfulness if you follow a systematic program of practice, so it becomes an integral part of your life.

The Latin expression *carpe diem* (meaning "seize the day") is an attitude that is often vividly present for those of us whose lives have been stripped down to essentials through suffering. I hope this book helps you seize all the moments of all the days in your life, with all the love in your heart.

PART I

*

A New Relationship
with Pain

CHAPTER 1

My Journey to the Present Moment

I had just turned twenty-three when I visited my parents' home in Wellington, New Zealand, for the Christmas holidays. Early on the morning of New Year's Day I was woken by the sound of a friend tapping at my window. He was driving to Auckland where I lived, and he offered me a lift. Still hungover from the previous night's celebrations, I slipped out quietly, leaving a note for my family, and fell asleep in the passenger seat. The next thing I knew, I was waking up in a mangled car, Tim's bloodied face beside me. He had fallen asleep at the wheel, and the car had hit a telephone pole beside the open road. My shoulder was hurting, my neck was hurting, my arm was hurting — and my back was hurting terribly. In addition to the pain, I remember the sounds in the car. In the background, behind Tim's wailing, was another noise. I gradually realized it was the sound of my own screams.

Six years before the car crash I had damaged my spine, fracturing a congenitally weak vertebra when I pulled someone out of a swimming pool during lifesaving practice. This led to months in a body cast, two major operations, and almost a year off school. Although I recovered to some extent, I still struggled to keep going in the face of physical pain. Now the car crash had smashed my weakened body. An ambulance took us to the hospital where I was told that I had a crushed collarbone, whiplash, a concussion, and a badly sprained wrist — as well as terrible back pain. It would be another two years before X-rays revealed that the accident had fractured an additional vertebra in the middle of my spine. Whatever chance I may have had to live without chronic pain was also destroyed, and pain, sometimes very intense, has been a continuous part of my experience for the last thirty years.

Chronic pain has been called the modern world's silent epidemic. The 2004 Pain in Europe study reported that one in seven people in the United Kingdom live with long-term persistent pain, and across Europe that's one in five.[1] It described the lives so many of us lead. Many people with pain feel isolated and desperate, and they believe they're a burden to their families, friends, and colleagues. Many have lost their jobs or been diagnosed with depression because of their pain, and for one in six that pain was sometimes so bad they wanted to die. A third reported that they experienced pain every minute of their lives, seven days a week. The story is the same in North America; eighty-three million Americans reported that pain affected their participation in work or other activities in 2000.[2]

This book is not a guide to the medical treatments that can help alleviate pain. It's about what happens if you're doing everything the doctors suggest and the pain is still there — which is the case for chronic pain sufferers. Is it possible to respond creatively, instead of falling into depression and despair? My own pain journey has been connected with the practice of mindful awareness and the teachings of Buddhism, which have a great deal to say about the experience of pain that's clear, practical, and relevant to the conditions we experience today. In recent years I've been sharing this approach with others who experience chronic pain, and friends have joined me in teaching what we call the "Breathworks" approach of mindfulness-based pain management. But before describing that approach, I want to relate an experience that followed the crash, which has informed my life ever since.

A few months after the accident I returned to work, but my whole spine was in pain, and I found working a physical and emotional strain. After two years of struggling I finally yielded to my mother's pleas to go back to the doctor. The consultant told me to go home and have two weeks of complete bed rest to see if things settled. So I went to bed, and having finally stopped my frenetic lifestyle, I collapsed. The years of overriding my body had taken their toll, and for months I didn't have the strength to get up.

It was a time of reckoning. Before the crash I'd been progressing in my career as a film and sound editor, sometimes working through the night when a deadline loomed. I loved my work, and it enabled me to maintain the lie — to myself as much as to others — that I was just as fit and active as I'd always been. My identity had been bound up with my job, but now I couldn't work.

After several months in bed I still wasn't improving physically, and another doctor offered to inject steroids into my spinal joints. After the shots I was in intense pain and had difficulty passing urine. Soon I was very ill, and my bladder stopped functioning completely. I was admitted to a hospital, put on a catheter, and transferred to the neurosurgical intensive–care ward for observation. I lay on my bed, bewildered: the other patients were recovering from brain hemorrhages and tumors— I'd never been around such ill people, and I was frightened.

After one procedure I had to sit upright for twenty-four hours to avoid complications. I hadn't sat up for months, but this time I had no choice. Throughout the long hours of the night I felt impaled on the edge of madness, and it seemed that two voices were speaking within me. One was saying, *I can't bear this. I'll go mad. There's no way I can endure this until morning.* But the other replied, *You have to bear it, you have no choice.* They argued incessantly, like a vice growing tighter every second. Suddenly, out of the chaos came something new. I felt a powerful clarity, and a third voice said, *You don't have to get through until morning. You only have to get through the present moment.*

Immediately, my experience was transformed. The tension torturing me opened into expansiveness as I realized the truth of what the third voice was saying. I knew, not intellectually but in the marrow of my bones, that life can only unfold one moment at a time. I saw that the present moment is always bearable, and I tasted the confidence this knowledge brings. Fear drained out of me and I relaxed.

As I sat propped up in the hospital bed that night, I realized much of my torment had grown out of fear of the future — the future moments of pain that I imagined stretching on until morning — rather than what I was actually experiencing in the present. Without understanding what had happened, I knew something extraordinary had broken through. It was a visceral experience that echoed like the reverberations of an earthquake through my body, feelings, and thoughts — and it tasted of freedom.

That long night of sitting was the axis on which my life has turned. What I saw that night broke through my defenses and showed me a completely different way of being. It was as if the compass of my life suddenly shifted and my habits, attitudes, and understanding have gradually been realigned. All the same, it has taken me many years of living with chronic pain to integrate those lessons into my daily experience in a way that's sustainable and practical. For some years I thought in terms of a simple dichotomy between pain (which was undesirable) and the absence of pain (desirable). Incredible as this might seem, I've learned that the chronic pain that I live with isn't really the problem. What really causes me to feel misery and distress is my *resistance* to suffering — the million ways that the mind and heart can say, *I don't want this to be happening to me.* That's what makes pain so very, very painful.

The change from an attitude of fighting to one of acceptance has been subtle and gradual, and I've been helped enormously by techniques that enabled me to steadily work with my states of mind: mindfulness and meditation. My first experience of meditation came when the hospital chaplain visited me, even though I didn't consider myself religious. He was a man of deep kindness who sat by my bed, held my hand, and guided me through a visualization in which he asked me to remember a time when I'd been happy. I took my mind back to holidays on New Zealand's South Island as a carefree teenager in love with the beauty of the high mountains. Through this, I made the profound discovery that, although my body was injured, my mind was still whole, and I could experience peace.

Leaving the hospital, I knew I couldn't return to my career in film. Somehow I had to find new values and goals, and I longed to recapture the peace I'd experienced when I relaxed into the present moment that night in intensive care and later when I meditated with the chaplain. Each day I spent hours lying on my bed listening to guided-meditation tapes and trying to make sense of things. Though my outer world was diminished, my inner world was flowering.

My journey took me to the Auckland Buddhist Center and eventually to Taraloka Women's Retreat Center in Shropshire, England, where I lived for five years. Gradually, I became more self-aware and more aware of the world around me. I learned to be with my experience, even if it was painful, and to inhabit my body with honesty and kindness.

Living with pain has changed me profoundly. Slowly I've been able to face the reality of my situation more often, and when I do, I find that this reality includes not only the pain and physical limitations of my body but also much that is subtle and beautiful. In resisting pain and trying to block it out, I'd also blocked out beauty, and in opening to the pain I opened the door to a wealth of emotions such as love, tenderness, and sensitivity. I've seen that life is bittersweet, and when I let go of expecting it to be either wonderful or awful and hold in an honest heart a sense of the delicate mixture of the two, I feel relaxed and open. Through facing and becoming sensitive to my own situation I've become a kinder, more tolerant person with far more sympathy for others.

PRIMARY AND SECONDARY SUFFERING

The approach outlined in this book grows from what I've learned in those years of trying to live with awareness while experiencing chronic pain. I've discovered that the experience of pain or suffering can be divided into two elements. First, there are the actual unpleasant sensations in the body in any given moment — I call this *"primary* suffering." And second, there are the myriad manifestations of resistance to those sensations that occur physically, mentally, and emotionally — often all at the same time — which I call *"secondary* suffering."

This distinction offers a key to living successfully with chronic pain because it provides a way for you to understand pain that allows you to make changes. It's easy to find yourself working with pain on the wrong level. If pain is an unavoidable fact of your life due to your circumstances and health, and you try to overcome or banish it, you're setting yourself up to fail. On the other hand, if you passively accept secondary suffering, you'll also experience unnecessary distress. But if you can distinguish the two levels of pain, you can then identify the habits of resistance that cause secondary suffering. Changing these habits reduces this aspect of your suffering, sometimes dramatically. You can find a way back to living creatively with a greater sense of being in control.

INGRID

Last autumn Ingrid's migraine headaches were getting worse and worse. When she heard me talk, she decided to walk toward her pain instead of resisting it. She stopped panicking and blaming herself and tried to develop kindness toward her pain instead. From that moment her migraines got much better.

MINDFULNESS-BASED PAIN MANAGEMENT AND THE BREATHWORKS APPROACH

I have never forgotten my experience as a young woman in the hospital when I felt so terribly alone, and after many years of meditation and mindfulness practice and thousands of hours of trying to be aware while sitting or lying in a painful body, eventually I felt I had something to offer others facing similar crises. I knew that mindfulness worked; I just needed to clarify how to offer it as a self-management program for others.

I learned from the example of Jon Kabat-Zinn, who established the Stress Reduction Clinic and Center for Mindfulness at the University of Massachusetts Medical Center in 1979 and developed mindfulness-based stress reduction (MBSR). Over sixteen thousand participants have been through this program, including many with chronic pain and illness.[3] In 2001 I attended one of his retreats and learned from Jon's presence and skill as a teacher, as well as from his experience of this work.

That same year I started my own work with a small pilot scheme and slowly formulated what became the Breathworks mindfulness–based pain management program. Along with my colleagues, Ratnaguna and Sona Fricker, I run courses for others living with pain, and more recently we've adapted the program for people dealing with stress or any other difficulty, such as anxiety, depression, or fatigue. We've trained others in delivering the program, and the Breathworks Community, though fairly new, runs activities in several countries as well as offers distance learning for people who can't get to a course or who are housebound. This book is another step in sharing what I've learned in these painful yet beautiful years.

My connection with mindfulness has come through my engagement with Buddhism, which explores mindfulness in great detail. Chapter 3 gives some background to Buddhism to suggest the context in which mindfulness practice originally developed. But you don't have to be a Buddhist to follow and understand the techniques and principles I introduce. Cultivating wise and kindly present–moment awareness is important within many philosophies,[4] and you can practice it whatever your religious convictions or background.

Mindfulness is also helpful whatever your condition. Many people with chronic pain haven't been given a clear diagnosis, and this can be very confusing, but a mindfulness-based approach is not concerned with the cause of your pain. What matters is your *experience* of pain, regardless of the diagnosis. Often a simple cause cannot be found, but it's always possible to find new ways to manage. The key is to pay attention to your experience in its wholeness instead of distracting yourself from it, even if this experience includes pain. This consciously developed awareness is called mindfulness, and the techniques in this book are aids to becoming more mindful. As your perceptions become more detailed and accurate, you can unravel the complex tapestry of pain and resistance, and clear space in your head and heart. This allows you to change your relationship with your primary suffering and reduce the secondary suffering that goes with chronic pain. It won't be straightforward, and resistance will reemerge many times, but with practice you'll learn to interrupt the cycle of tension, reaction, and suffering, and replace it with kindness, awareness, and choice.

Mindfulness can be practiced alongside other treatments you may be receiving, and I encourage you to get all the help you can from both conventional and complementary therapies — if that seems appropriate. I've worked with people who haven't had pain for long and others who have experienced it for decades. We've had people in our courses with terminal cancer who have used mindfulness alongside their chemotherapy, and others who simply wanted to find ways to make the best of the time they had left. The only requirement is that you're motivated and prepared to engage with the practices and methods outlined in this book.

When I meet people in my courses I always tell them that I believe their suffering is real (which can be a great relief to hear) and encourage them to start taking responsibility right away. You don't need to wait for the doctors to finish their treatments or investigations before you practice mindfulness. In truth, there's no time to waste, and there's no need to wait. You can start now. What are you waiting for?

CHAPTER 2

What Is Pain?

Before outlining the Breathworks program in detail, it's worth pausing to ask if this mindfulness-based approach fits in with the modern medical understanding of pain. Does it make sense to work with chronic pain at the level of reactions and resistance? Answering this means looking at an even more basic question that many people with chronic pain never hear properly discussed: "What is pain?"

The commonsense view is that pain is a result of damage to the body. In the seventeenth century the French philosopher René Descartes developed a "rope-pull" model of pain. Just as pulling a rope in a church tower rings the bell, Descartes thought that tissue damage in the body is a tug that causes the sensation of pain in the brain. For centuries following Descartes, Western doctors regarded pain as a sensation that could be explained by neurology. The intensity of the pain was thought to be directly proportionate to the degree of damage to the body, which would mean that if different people had the same injury, they would experience the same pain. If no obvious physical cause could be found, often the patient would be accused of malingering.

In the last half-century, views of pain changed dramatically as scientists discovered the extent to which it involves the whole person — the mind as well as the body — and research using sophisticated new methods shows just how complex pain really is. The leading professional body of pain specialists, the International Association for the Study of Pain (IASP), has come up with a definition of pain that most health professionals use when assessing physical pain problems. They call it "an unpleasant sensory and emotional experience associated with actual or potential tissue damage, or which is described in terms of such damage."[1] They add that "pain is always subjective."[2]

The key point is that pain is an *experience*. As anyone with chronic pain knows, that experience is deeply personal, and scientists are finding that the way you experience pain is influenced by many factors in your life. Emotions, beliefs, and attitudes that are influential in your society and culture, as well as past experiences, all play a role in how you perceive the experience we label "pain[3]." In this book I'll use the term "pain" very broadly to describe any unpleasant experience that has a physical dimension, whether caused by disease, injury, stress, or emotion, and I'll introduce ways of living with the experience of pain regardless of its cause. I also want to describe some of the physiological mechanisms that cause pain as modern research describes them because I've found that understanding these helps me avoid making my pain worse with anxiety.

ACUTE AND CHRONIC PAIN

Pain can be divided into two main categories: acute and chronic.

Acute pain is what you experience in the short term following an injury. If you stub a toe or touch something hot, you'll feel an acute pain that is a direct consequence of a pain signal sent from the injured muscles, bones, ligaments, or skin. This pain is part of the body's built-in alarm system, signaling it's under attack, and it tells you that you need to take care of the injured area to allow it to heal. You'll probably see inflammation such as a bruise, swelling, or blister, and feel pain at the site of the injury. Following an injury, all sorts of chemical and physical responses are set off in the affected cells and tissues that begin healing the damage. Most healing is completed within six weeks, and acute pain usually reduces over this period, too.

Nearly all injured tissues are fully healed within six months. Acute pain also arises without obvious injury, as with a stomachache after overeating, or the headache that comes with a hangover.

Chronic pain, also called *persistent* or *long-term* pain, is pain that has lasted for three months or more[4] — sometimes it can continue for decades. The word "chronic" is often misunderstood to mean "severe." (English people sometimes say, "Oh, my back hurts something chronic!") But it actually means long-term. Chronic pain sometimes develops after an injury and persists, often inexplicably, after tissue healing has taken place. Or it may start for no obvious or specific reason. If the pain remains even when there's no continuing physical damage, the experience of pain becomes a medical problem in its own right and is often known as "chronic-pain syndrome."

Experts differ in how they talk about different kinds of chronic pain,[5] but they agree that it's complex and multifaceted. Some pain is caused by obvious tissue damage that persists over time — for example, in the case of arthritis and cancer. The pain is caused by continuing physical processes at the area of disease or joint degeneration, and there seems to be a clear cause of the unpleasant sensations.

Neuropathic pain occurs in the nervous system rather than being prompted by tissue damage, and it can be confusing — often normal medical tests don't show any obvious cause. Sometimes neuropathic pain is caused by damage or injury to the nerves, the spinal cord, or the brain, but sometimes pain is felt even when there's no damage or when healing has completed at the site of the injury. Doctors think the nervous system responds to the experience of pain by increasing its capacity to process pain signals, just as a computer devotes extra circuits and memory to an important task. The central nervous system can then become oversensitized so that a little pain feels far worse. Another analogy is that the nervous system is like an amplifier of pain sensations. When you develop chronic pain it's as if the amplifier has been turned up high.

Neuropathic pain can also take the form of unusual sensations such as electric shocks, the sensation of water, burning, or distorted perceptions of the body. I frequently have a feeling of burning on the soles of my feet or the sensation of hot wax being dripped onto my shin even though there's no tissue damage in those parts of my body. Another example of neuropathic pain is phantom-limb pain, when pain persists in a limb after it has been amputated. In each case, the sensation of pain is produced by nerves that have been damaged or whose signals have become confused in some way. An engineer might say that neuropathic pain such as this is an electrical rather than a mechanical fault.

The main thing to understand about neuropathic pain is that it's *real,* and when it is severe it can be absolutely devastating. You may think you're making it up if there's no apparent mechanical cause, but it's increasingly recognized in the medical world that neuropathic pain is a cause of suffering in its own right, and it can be very unpleasant.

In many cases, chronic pain has a variety of causes: it may result from mechanical problems due to a disease such as arthritis, from muscle strains because of poor posture, or from the wear and tear that comes with age; it may also be produced by an oversensitized nervous system.

These scientific descriptions of the causes of chronic pain reflect my experience of it. I experience mechanical weaknesses and strains due to old injuries, nerve damage, and surgery, and I also experience oversensitivity — as if pain has become a default setting in my nervous system. Sometimes I think of this chronic pain as completely useless "white noise" that's constantly present in the background of my life: it's like being trapped in a room with a radio that's tuned off the station and produces constant hissing, crackling, and humming.

CURRENT RESEARCH INTO CHRONIC PAIN

A great deal of research is taking place into the experience of pain using modern scanning and imaging techniques. In recent years, imaging techniques such as positron emission tomography (PET) and functional magnetic resonance imaging (fMRI) have for the first time enabled scientists to scan the brain while doing active experiments. They can see pictures of the brain at the very moment when a person is having a painful stimulus, and results show the perception of pain is very complicated. The brain makes sense of stimuli from the body by creating an image or representation that scientists call the *neuromatrix*. The brain compares incoming signals with what's expected, using the neuromatrix as a guide in identifying their location, quality, and the degree of threat the signals offer while ignoring familiar sensations such as the contact of clothes and the skin. But pain isn't a normal experience so it grabs the brain's attention, overriding other claims. This, then, affects the perception and discrimination of other sensations and emotions, and scans even show changes in the brain of someone living with chronic pain that are associated with the heightened sensitivity they feel.

This more complex understanding of pain challenges many assumptions. For example, you'd think that if a person has back pain, detailed MRI scans would allow doctors to see the cause of the problem. In fact, in a study where a number of people *without* back pain were scanned, 64 percent had disk abnormalities in the spine,[6] while in another study of people *with* back pain, 85 percent had no obvious damage.[7] Research also shows huge individual variation in pain perception. Two individuals given the same pain stimulus while being monitored in the scanner can show vastly different brain activity.[8]

One well-established view of pain is the gate control theory developed in the 1960s by Patrick Wall — a world-renowned neuroscientist who specialized in studying pain — and his collaborator Ronald Melzack. [9] They suggested that there are "gates" in the nerve junctions, spinal cord, and the brain's pain centers. For you to experience pain, these gates need to be opened, which is what happens when a healthy person is injured. Pain messages are a signal to protect that part of the body that helps it to heal. The gates can also close, which means pain is reduced or stopped. Again, this is what happens in the case of a healthy person when healing is complete.

Opening and closing these gates is a complex process that is affected by emotional states, mental activity, and where your attention is focused. Whether the brain expects pain or is primed to detect any damage or strain also has an impact. When you expect pain, the pain pathways (or gates) open, so the brain doesn't miss anything—and the pain experience is amplified. People with chronic pain commonly report they manage some pain effectively, but a sudden, unexpected increase in pain feels much worse because of the fear that it's caused by new damage. The anxiety causes the gates to open or to stay open longer.

Many researchers are searching for ways to close the gates in people living with chronic pain, so their nervous system can return to normal functioning. Mindfulness training may be one way to do this because it calms the whole mental, physical, emotional, and nervous system, allowing it to return to a state of balance.

WORKING WITH PAIN

The view of pain that's emerging from research includes the mind, the body, and the environment. As Patrick Wall wrote:

> Pure pain is never detected as an isolated sensation. Pain is always accompanied by emotion and meaning so that each pain is unique to the individual. The word "pain" is used to group together a class of combined sensory-emotional events. The class contains many different types of pain, each of which is a personal, unique experience for the person who suffers.[10]

This growing awareness of the complexity of pain shows doctors that treating it involves the whole of a person's experience. The *biopsychosocial* model of pain, widely used in chronic pain management, suggests that the biological, psychological, and social aspects of an individual's life all influence the way that person deals with pain. This has led doctors to develop multifaceted pain management programs — intensive courses, often run in hospitals, that offer in-depth help in managing the many ways in which pain has affected a person's life. Input is often available from a range of professionals, such as physiotherapists, anesthetists, occupational therapists, and psychologists.

Mindfulness-based pain management is one such program. It combines the scientific view of pain with an understanding of the nature of experience that comes from the experience of meditation and mindfulness. These practices have ancient roots in the Buddhist tradition, but they augment scientific understanding in practical ways by offering methods to respond constructively to pain. The next chapter explores what mindfulness is and how it works, using a story told by the Buddha himself.

CHAPTER 3

The Two Arrows

The story of the two arrows was first taught by the Buddha, who lived in northern India 2,600 years ago and spent his early adult life investigating his mind through contemplation and meditation. When he was thirty-five he gained a state that Buddhists call "enlightenment" or "awakening," which he described as a complete mental and emotional liberation that brought a deep understanding of human experience. He spent the rest of his life passing on his insights, and the methods he taught to train the hearts and minds of people form the basis of the Buddhist tradition.

Although generally described as a religion, Buddhism can also be seen simply as an approach to life. It's pragmatic and experiential rather than being concerned, for example, with belief in a creator god. Buddhist reflection and meditation involve careful examination of the exact processes of moment-to-moment experience, and Buddhist philosophy and practice are attracting growing interest from psychologists and medical practitioners in the West.[1]

The Buddha's teaching is concerned with coming to terms with suffering. The starting point is that suffering is an inherent part of human experience and at the heart of our predicament. No one wants to suffer, and yet, in reality, everyone experiences some degree of pain at one time or another. The Buddha suggests that rather than being driven solely by the desire to eliminate or avoid suffering, the wise person learns to *change his or her relationship with it*. Of course, some pain can be eased, and it's sensible to do so—eating when you're hungry or taking a painkiller to relieve a headache, for example. But chronic, intractable pain or a terminal illness (like the existential pain that is also part of the human condition) cannot be easily removed, and the wise person knows a deeper solution is needed.

In the text that relates the story of the two arrows, the Buddha gives practical guidance in changing your relationship with pain. Asked to describe the difference between the response of a wise person and that of an ordinary person to pain, the Buddha uses the analogy of being pierced by an arrow:

> When an ordinary person experiences a painful bodily feeling
> they worry, agonize and feel distraught. Then they feel two types
> of pain — one physical and one mental. It's as if this person was
> pierced by an arrow, and then immediately afterwards by a second
> arrow, and they experience the pain of two arrows.[2]

This image describes my own experience of pain. I have an unpleasant feeling in my body — in my case, it's back pain. This is the first arrow. But immediately it seems I'm assailed by fear, sorrow, anger, anxiety, and similar distressing emotions. This is the second arrow, and it means that on top of the physical pain, I now experience a mass of additional suffering. In fact, it frequently feels as if a whole volley of second arrows assails me! Grief and sorrow are often appropriate responses to pain, but even these healthy emotional responses become more complex and problematic if they dominate you. They become not only a response to pain but causes of additional pain in themselves, as the Buddha explains:

> Having been touched by that painful feeling, they resist and resent
> it. They harbor aversion to it, and this underlying tendency of
> resistance and resentment toward that painful feeling comes to
> obsess the mind.[3]

It seems the human mind has been following the same well-worn grooves for millennia. The second arrow comes because you respond by trying to push away the first arrow—the physical pain. Paradoxically, the effort of resisting pain means your energy gets tied up with it until the "underlying tendency of resistance" becomes a habit that you revert to again and again without knowing why. In my own experience, and from what I've learned from others who have attended the Breathworks course, this *resistance* to pain is the major cause of suffering and distress. It's what causes you to be pierced by the second arrow—and the same is true of any intractable difficulty, be it physical or mental.

The Buddha now goes into more detail about how this resistance makes us behave:

Touched by that painful feeling, the ordinary person delights in compulsive distraction, often through seeking pleasure. Why is that? Because compulsive distraction is the only way they know to escape from painful feeling. This underlying tendency of craving for distraction comes to obsess the mind.[4]

When I first heard this I didn't agree, as my main response to pain is to push things away rather than to seek pleasure to replace it. Instead of reaching for the chocolates, I'm more likely to pick a fight. But on deeper reflection I realized I was picking fights because, perverse though it might be, I found having an argument more enjoyable than experiencing the pain. When I revert to distraction in this way, whatever form it takes, I erect a barrier that separates me from unpleasant experience. It seems sensible at the time, but it creates more and more layers of resistance: as if I think I can escape my own shadow if I run away from myself fast enough.

If you look at your own experience you'll probably find favorite versions of compulsive distraction that you revert to whenever you try to escape from painful feelings — obvious "pleasures" such as ciga-rettes, chocolates, recreational drugs, alcohol, and shopping, or more subtle ones like arguments or obsessively engaging in activities such as cleaning or tidying.

It's important to realize the Buddha isn't suggesting that all pleasure is bad. Living with mindfulness and awareness, life actually becomes lighter, freer, more fun, and much more satisfying. Indeed, mindful or aware "distraction" — consciously taking your mind off things — can sometimes be a useful strategy when living with pain. When the Buddha mentions pleasure-seeking, he means the blind and driven ways we compulsively look for distraction and entrench habits of unawareness and avoidance. Just as resistance quickly becomes a habit, compulsive distraction soon turns into obsession.

I have many habitual ways of distracting myself from my back pain. In addition to arguing, I find myself restlessly surfing the Internet, wandering around the house like a caged animal, making endless cups of tea, and finding myself surveying the contents of the fridge without quite knowing how I got there. All these states are accompanied by tension and strain, and it can be a tremendous effort to stop whatever I'm doing and come back to a more whole and aware sense of myself. As the Buddha explains, these compul-sive habits of avoidance are stressful:

> Being overwhelmed and dominated by pain (through resistance and compulsive distraction), the ordinary person is joined with suffering and stress.[5]

The battle with pain, which is lived out through resistance, aversion, and obsession, compounds suffering and stress. I become "joined with" my pain and my reactions to it, even fettered to it. A fetter is a chain fastened round the ankle, and when I'm compulsively reacting to my pain — either through avoidance or obsession — I really do feel as if I'm chained. Before I know it, my whole experience seems like a dense web of conflicting pulls and tendencies. To summarize:

- First comes the experience of pain — the basic unpleasant sensations. This is what the Buddha called the first arrow and what I have termed *primary suffering.*
- Then you respond to the pain with aversion, resistance, and resentment.
- Next, you seek to escape from pain by getting caught up in compulsive distractions and avoidance strategies.
- Ironically, in your attempts to escape the pain you become stuck in a troubled state until, finally, you're joined or fettered to suffering and stress, and this dominates your life and obsesses your mind. It is what the Buddha called the second arrow and what I describe as *secondary suffering.*

BLOCKING AND DROWNING

When I examine my own experience in more detail and talk to others with chronic pain, I see recurring patterns in how my resistance is lived out in day-to-day behavior. These patterns can be grouped into the two tendencies of *blocking* and *drowning.* I think you'll find your own particular recipe of avoidance strategies fits into one of these categories.

Blocking: Obvious Resistance and Avoidance

When you run away from something you don't like, you can feel restless, brittle, and driven, as if you can't stop; you get caught in addictions as you attempt to block out the pain — alcohol, cigarettes, recreational drugs, shopping, chocolate, work, talking, sleeping, and so on. Every time the pain breaks back into your experience, you reach for more of your chosen addiction and before you know it, you're spinning in the hamster wheel of avoidance, anxiety, and panic.

Drowning: Obsession and Feeling Overwhelmed

Alternatively, you may feel preoccupied and overwhelmed by your pain. You lose perspective and feel as if you're drowning in it, that it's the only thing in your experience. You may also feel exhausted and depressed and find it hard to function. It may not be obvious that a sense of being dominated by pain is a form of resistance to it, but as with blocking, a drowning reaction grows from an underlying desire for your experience to be different from the way it really is.

❊

One common pattern is to run away from the pain, hectically pursuing avoidance strategies to block it out. You can keep this up for a while but there's a cost: it's very tiring and eventually your capacity to continue running is used up. Your defenses are breached, you feel exhausted, and the pain comes crashing back into your awareness, often with a ferocious intensity. Now you tend to swing to the other extreme and collapse, feeling overwhelmed. As the pain dominates your experience you'll probably lose perspective and forget there's anything in life apart from pain: it can almost feel as if you have *become* that pain. After a time, your resources and energy recover a little, and you become more active again. For a while you manage to feel more balanced, but before you know it you're back into patterns of avoidance and compulsive distraction, accompanied by the familiar whirring of the hamster wheel. And so it goes on, in a depressingly familiar cycle.

These tendencies express themselves differently in different people. Most of us living with chronic health problems flip-flop between blocking and drowning. You might go through a cycle with big extremes over a long period, or you may experience the two poles within shorter cycles that happen several times a day, even within moments.

PRIMARY SUFFERING
(First arrow)

CHRONIC PAIN/ILLNESS
(in the sense of basic unpleasant sensations)

RESISTANCE

SECONDARY SUFFERING
(Second arrow)

BLOCKING	DROWNING
• Hardening against unpleasant sensations	• Feeling overwhelmed by unpleasant sensations
• Restlessness	• Exhaustion
• Inability to "stop"	• Physical inactivity leading to loss of function, weakening of muscles, etc.
• Feeling driven	• Giving up

• Addictions of all kinds. e.g.
  – food
  – cigarettes
  – alcohol
  – recreational drugs
  – excessive talking
  – excessive working
	• Lack of interest, vagueness

• Being emotionally brittle and edgy	• Being emotionally dull and passive
• Anxiety	• Depression
• Anger and irritability	• Self-pity and victim mentality
• Denial	• Tendency to catastrophize and loss of perspective
• Being "in head" not "in body"	• Dominated by physical experience

• Overly controlling	• Loss of initiative
	  – withdrawal
	  – isolation

FIGURE 1: THE WISE ARROWS

THE WISE RESPONSE

According to the Buddha, there's an alternative response to painful bodily feelings, which is that of a wise person:

> *When a wise person experiences a painful bodily feeling, they*
> *don't worry, agonize, or feel distraught, and they feel physical*
> *pain but not mental pain. It's as if this person was pierced by an*
> *arrow, but a second arrow didn't follow this, so they only experi-*
> *ence the pain of a single arrow.*[6]

Even a wise person, at peace with him- or herself and who lives in harmony with the human condition, still experiences the first arrow. Suffering is an inescapable part of experience: if this isn't outright physical pain it might be the ache of separation from people dear to you, finding yourself in situations that are unpleasant for you, or the difficulties that come with age. A friend recently told me that when his children were babies he felt huge love for them, but he also experienced the pain of knowing that life would throw difficulties in their way. Their newborn perfection would be knocked about, and there was nothing he could do to prevent it beyond providing care and shelter. I'm sure every parent knows this aching, painful love; there's no way to protect your children from the first arrow.

The inevitability of suffering is obvious when you think about it, but it's surprising how deeply we resist this fact. For many years I saw my back pain as a sign of failure and tried unrealistically to find cures instead of taking responsibility for my reactions to the pain. When I saw that pain was a natural part of life I felt relief. I realized my lack of acceptance was far more painful than the back pain itself.

The difference in a wise person's response to suffering, the Buddha says, is that they don't try to escape painful feelings by resisting them and feeling aversion, or by compulsively seeking distraction. Therefore:

> *The wise person is not joined with suffering and stress. This is the difference between the wise person and the ordinary person.*[7]

The Buddha suggests we can move toward acceptance of primary suffering and avoid secondary suffering by being like the wise person who "discerns and understands" his or her feelings "as they are actually present." In other words, we must pay attention to our experience as it really is without trying to block it out or feeling overwhelmed.

How Mindfulness Helps

Cultivating this wise response may sound daunting or even unrealistic if you're living with pain. It's easy to get locked into aversion and distraction, to relate to pain as a fixed and hard "thing" — a monster lurking in the shadows that dominates your life because you fear it. That's where mindfulness comes in. The awareness you can develop through mindfulness is steady, calm, and kind, and it's subtle and precise enough for you to notice the different elements of an experience. Paying attention to a painful sensation, for example, allows you to investigate it, to explore its texture, and to see it for what it is rather than what you imagine it to be. You can make surprising discoveries, such as finding that the sensations you identify as "my pain" are continually changing; there may even be pleasant sensations or feelings alongside them. You may also notice that in addition to the painful sensations, you experience physical tension, distressing and angry thoughts about your pain, or escapist fantasies and restlessness, and you may feel irritable, frustrated, or upset.

If you can catch this resistance before it overwhelms you, you have the chance to relax into a broader awareness. The key is to allow the feelings to arise and pass away, moment by moment, with an attitude of receptivity and openness. This creates an opening in the dense web of habits, a moment of choice that offers a tiny chance to make a new beginning in each moment by interrupting the usual cascade of reactions. This is the battleground of awareness, because habitual impulses can be compelling, and it takes courage to resist them — but it's also the point of freedom in which you can find a key to living with joy, confidence, and creativity.

ALAN

Following a car accident, Alan had severe leg pain. When he first attended a Breathworks course, he was overwhelmed by the pain and felt it had destroyed his life. But when he investigated his pain directly, he experienced it as a wave of sensations flowing up his leg that were continually changing and not nearly as bad as he feared. He also noticed pleasant elements alongside the pain, such as the softness of his breath and the warmth of his hands. His face lit up as he told the class that, for the first time in years, he felt some freedom in how he related to his pain.

Breaking the Cycle

Mindfulness is also the key to breaking the cycle of blocking and drowning. It means you can catch yourself whenever you find you are tipping into either extreme, and choose to behave differently. If you're blocking, you are able to soften the resistance and include the pain in your field of awareness; if you're drowning, you can broaden your perspective to encompass elements of your experience other than the pain.

I've realized that I can maintain the blocking part of the cycle for months at a time. As such, I become more and more hardened to the pain in my body and more and more brittle and driven in my interactions, as if a powerful force is pushing me to avoid relaxing. At such times I genuinely believe my pain isn't so bad and I'm coping, even though my friends tell me I'm not very pleasant to be around! Eventually I reach a state of exhaustion; common sense prevails, and I'm forced to rest my weary body. At this point I sometimes experience a flare-up of pain as I feel the consequences of being harsh toward my body. It's sobering to realize that I've been bullying it through the day.

When I finally recover my energy and emerge from this state of collapse, I often experience a beautiful softness and openness, as if my perceptions have been cleansed and I can balance living a rich, full life with treating my body with care and consideration. This is the point of greatest potential and greatest danger—when I feel an urgent motivation to change, but my habits are waiting to pounce. It's the moment to be mindful! If I'm able to stay with this broad, deep, kindly, and yet proactive sense of myself, I can avoid the second arrow. But if I don't take care, I quickly tip back into blocking and drowning.

As my mindfulness practice has deepened over the years, the extremes of my pain reactions have become smaller. Although I still alternate between blocking and drowning, I catch the tipping points much earlier. This is entirely because I practice mindfulness. I'm not claiming to have mastered my reactions to my chronic pain completely, but I've learned that every moment contains an opportunity for choice as long as I remain aware, notice my unhelpful habits, and stand firm against them. Gradually, I am finding that it's possible to experience a sense of creativity and freedom within the struggles of everyday life while living with pain.

Acceptance

Although turning your attention toward your pain may seem scary, people in our courses often say that it's a tremendous relief. For those of us with chronic conditions, *changing our relationship* with them is the very best medicine. Being locked in a battle with your pain is exhausting, and it reinforces the sense that something is deeply wrong in your life. Letting go of resistance and learning to stay with what's actually happening can be a homecoming for the heart. This attitude of acceptance is well expressed by the Christian serenity prayer, which echoes the lesson of the two arrows:

> *Lord, give me the serenity to accept the things I cannot change*
> *[the first arrow];*
> *the courage to change the things I can*
> *[the second arrow];*
> *and the wisdom to know the difference*
> *[mindfulness is the tool that can help you do this].*

*

PART II

Mindfulness and Healing

CHAPTER 4

Exploring Mindfulness

The whole path of mindfulness is this:
whatever you are doing, be aware of it.

DIPA MA, BUDDHIST MEDITATION TEACHER¹

The best way to get a sense of mindfulness is through experiencing it directly. Here's a short exercise that will give you a taste of mindfulness right now. (You can download an audio version of this exercise from soundstrue.com/burch.)

MINDFULNESS EXERCISE

Adopt a comfortable posture and notice how your body feels. What physical sensations are you experiencing at this moment? Maybe you feel pressure between your pelvis and the chair you're sitting on. What does this feel like? For a few moments just be open to any sensations in your body.

Now take a moment to listen to any sounds you're hearing. Observe their quality, register, and volume and how you're responding to them. You may notice an automatic tendency to try to identify their source, but see if you can suspend that for a moment and just notice the sounds as sounds. If you're in a very quiet environment, then notice the silence.

Now notice your breath. What does it feel like? What parts of your body move as you breathe, and how many different movements can you feel? Is it pleasant or unpleasant to be in touch with your breathing?

Now allow your awareness to be with your emotions. What is the broad tone of your emotional experience? Are you happy, content, sad, irritated, or calm? Or is it hard to be sure what you are feeling?

Notice any thoughts that are passing through your mind. You can ask yourself, *What am I thinking?* Rest your attention on your thoughts for a few moments.

Now spend a few moments resting quietly with the sensations of the breath in your body and let any thoughts, sounds, and feelings come and go. There's no need to look for a special experience. Simply notice what is actually happening, moment by moment.

If you've been able to engage with this short practice, you've just had an experience of mindfulness. Perhaps this may seem very ordinary, but the implications of bringing awareness to your experience in this way are immense. It means you can move from autopilot (being driven by habits as you drift from one thing to the next) to experiencing life as a stream of creative possibilities and choice. You can only choose your response to things if you're aware of what's happening, so mindfulness training consists of becoming aware, over and over again. This awareness allows those of us living with pain and illness to be with our primary suffering in an accepting and uncluttered way and to interrupt the habits that cause secondary suffering.

The difference between being on autopilot and being mindful is like the comparison between being asleep and awake. Mindfulness, after all, is sometimes described as *wakefulness* or alertness. Imagine what life would be like if every moment you continually felt alert, alive, and awake; wise, clear, and receptive; and able to engage with, and appreciate, the world around you. This is a wonderful state to aim for, but when you did the mindfulness exercise you may have noticed that it was hard to keep your attention on one thing at a time. Most people find that the mind likes to wander — it almost seems to have a will of its own. So mindfulness practice involves continually calling the mind back from wherever it has wandered.

You might think that every time your mind wanders you've failed to be mindful. A much more helpful attitude is to see every moment in which you notice directly what's happening as a moment of success, no matter how fleeting it may have been. Mindfulness training means experiencing more and more of these "magic moments" until, eventually, awareness flows through the whole of your life.

THE ROOTS OF MINDFULNESS

The origins of mindfulness lie in the ancient teachings and practices of Buddhism.[2] Over the past thirty years, more and more Westerners, such as those led by Jon Kabat-Zinn, have adapted mindfulness to secular settings to help deal with the strains of modern life. At Breathworks we've continued this exploration and developed our own applications of mindfulness.

To practice mindfulness is to live in the moment, notice what is happening, and make choices about how you respond to your experience rather than being driven by habitual reactions. Kabat-Zinn describes it as "a particular way of paying attention: on purpose, in the present moment, and nonjudgmentally."[3] He and his colleagues draw out three key aspects:

- Mindfulness is *intentional*. It includes a sense of purpose that enables us to make choices and act with awareness, helping life to unfold in a creative way.
- Mindfulness is *experiential,* allowing us to focus on present-moment awareness based on accurate and direct perception.
- Mindfulness is *nonjudgmental*. It allows us to see things as they actually are in the present moment without automatically making harsh value judgments. We definitely

need intelligent discernment of our experience just to make our way through the day, but it's important to distinguish this from the "habit of judging that winds up functioning as an irrational tyrant that can never be satisfied."[4]

Mindfulness also involves a rich emotional awareness and could equally be described as "heartfulness,"[5] or compassionate and kindly awareness. Mind and heart are two doorways into the experience of awareness, and both are gradually transformed as your practice of mindfulness deepens. I like to describe mindfulness as *becoming intimate with experience*. If you're caring for a loved one or a child, it isn't enough to pay attention in a cold and clinical way. With mindfulness, our relationship to our impulses and responses includes love, care, tenderness, and interest. That means deeply inhabiting the richness of the moment in an embodied and authentic way — especially important if you're in pain. You can only look at life with honesty and integrity and be open to its painful and pleasurable sides if you have a soft and open heart; it takes courage to face the demon of pain instead of frantically running away from it.

Though rooted in Buddhist meditation, mindfulness also has a long ancestry in the West. The Stoic philosophers of ancient Greece prized the qualities of attention and concentration on the present moment. According to the historian Pierre Hadot, their practice involved "continuous vigilance and presence of mind, self-consciousness which never sleeps." Like the Buddhists, the Greeks believed that "by encouraging concentration on the minuscule present moment which is always bearable and controllable, attention increases your vigilance," and such attention enables you to see "the infinite value of each instant, and causes you to accept each moment of existence from the viewpoint of the universal law of the cosmos."[6]

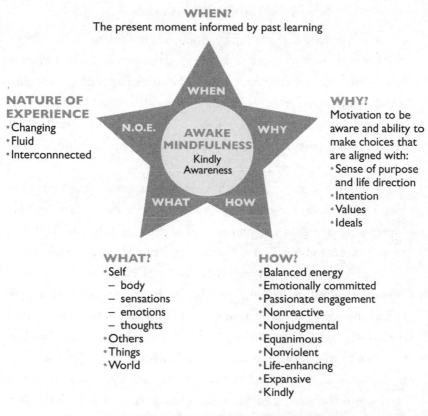

FIGURE 2: MINDFULNESS STAR

EXPLORING THE NATURE OF MINDFULNESS

We can get a fuller sense of mindfulness by considering it in five ways, as illustrated by figure 2: The Mindfulness Star.

- When can I be aware?
- Why should I want to be aware?
- How am I aware?
- What am I aware of?
- What is the nature of what I'm aware of?

When Can I Be Aware?

The simple answer is that I can be aware, or mindful, in each moment. We all spend much of our time dwelling on the past and imagining the future, but what we can affect directly is what's happening right now. If you're awake to each unfolding moment rather than lost in regrets and fantasies, you can be fully alive to everything in yourself, other people, and the world around you. The only opportunity for wise action is now — and now and now.

Mindfulness is sometimes defined as "bare attention."[7] This suggests that being mindful means you just have your experience without suppressing elements you find painful or reacting to them.[8] It brings about a broad and equanimous receptivity that allows you to see things just as they are and creates conditions for creativity and initiative. You'll also notice your automatic responses before they're expressed in behavior, and in that small window of awareness it's possible to hold negative reactions in check. Then you can choose to steer yourself in the direction you want to go, instead of being trapped helplessly in compulsive habits. If you notice an impulse to lash out at others when you are in pain, you can instead choose to take some deep breaths and remain silent. You can use that pause to see things from another person's point of view.

It's easy to imagine the present as something isolated from past and future. In fact, one of the Indian words for mindfulness (*sati*) comes from a root meaning "to remember," suggesting that awareness of the present is closely connected with recalling the past. You can only understand the experiences you're having right now if you learn from the past. For example, you might have learned that exercising is helpful if you wake up stiff, or you may realize that the particular pain you're feeling is one you're familiar with, so you needn't panic. You may also have learned from bitter experience that speaking harshly causes pain to yourself and others. The past is a compass that helps you make sense of the present and choose wisely in responding to it.[9]

Mindfulness also allows you to "remember" to be awake in the present moment. You need to "remember" continually to be present, rather than getting lost in daydreams about the past or the future. If you're fully present in this moment, it will also be easier to recollect the content of this present-moment experience in the future; that may mean something simple such as remembering where you put the car keys, or it could mean reconnecting to a deeper sense of moral and ethical continuity, which means you needn't keep relearning the same lessons.

Why Should I Want to Be Aware?

In addition to learning from the past, your present actions lead to consequences in the future, so it's not enough to simply be aware. You also need to make sense of your experience — and mindfulness brings an intelligent, responsive awareness to your ever-changing conditions.[10] An important aspect of mindfulness is motivation and intention: what's important to you in your life and where do you want to go? [11] If you have mindfulness in this sense, you know what you're doing *and* why you're doing it. [12]

If your dreams and aspirations are realistic, they *can* be realized if you make choices in each moment that are in line with your values. Every action has consequences, and it's up to you whether or not they're beneficial. If you decide to stay in bed rather than get up and begin to move your body, this will have consequences. In the short term things may feel easier, but ultimately, sleeping your way through life will be unsatisfying. Trying to become more aware also has consequences; choosing wakefulness, even if this includes elements that are painful, means you feel much more alive and engaged. It's up to you. This principle is simple, but its implications are astounding.

Making choices means being the master of your actions. Sometimes there seem to be hundreds of selves within each of us. One moment you want one thing, the next something else entirely. Mindfulness brings these contradictory tendencies into the light of awareness, allowing the heart and mind to become integrated, collected, and whole, rather than distracted and scattered. Then you can make choices that grow from all aspects of yourself.

How Am I Aware?

The quality of your awareness is important if your practice of mindfulness is to be sustainable and balanced. If your awareness is too relaxed, you'll slip into distraction and vagueness, whereas trying too hard simply leads to headaches and tension. The balanced approach is to be alert, awake, and emotionally engaged, while remaining relaxed and receptive. The Buddhist teacher Sangharakshita describes this engagement as "an iridescent . . . emotionally committed awareness."[13]

Effort is important, but when applied mindfully its quality is gentle, open, and receptive. If you lose something important, then fret and struggle to remember where you left it, you'll find that the more you strain, the less you remember. But if you put the problem aside and let your mind relax, suddenly you remember where it is! A good image for this balanced effort is a mother watching her child in an enclosed playground. She's alert because she's concerned for the child's safety, but she's also relaxed because her child is in a protected area. In the Buddhist tradition, paying attention with mindfulness is compared to the way an elephant looks at something. It turns with its whole body, not just its head, and gives full, complete attention.[14]

As Jon Kabat-Zinn points out, mindfulness is also nonjudgmental and nonreactive. Many of us automatically judge ourselves harshly: *I'm no good at anything. I'm useless. I shouldn't be feeling sad. I should be able to manage my pain better.* Or you feel guilty when you're happy or successful or get something you think you don't deserve. But these are all value judgments heaped on top of experience. With mindfulness you notice these reactions and find the most creative way to act. As Jon Kabat-Zinn says, "Mindfulness includes an affectionate, compassionate quality within the attending, a sense of openhearted, friendly presence and interest."[15]

MINDFULNESS REFLECTION

Remember a time when you were happily absorbed in an activity—maybe painting, playing music, gazing at a beautiful sunset, cooking, or working at an enjoyable task. When you're fully mindful you no longer feel awkward, self-conscious, and separate—you feel at one with the activity. You feel that you dwell in a timeless present moment, and your body and its senses and the activity become part of a harmonious whole.

Mindfulness is always seen in the Buddhist tradition as "wholesome."[16] It's a special, nonviolent, and life-enhancing sort of awareness that helps one move *toward* life rather than contracting away from it, and it is aligned with values such as openness, kindliness, and release.

What Am I Aware Of?

Mindfulness means being aware of everything in your experience—yourself, other people, and the world around you—but a traditional guide called the *Satipatthana Sutta,* translated variously as "presences of mindfulness," "attending with mindfulness," or "foundations of mindfulness," suggests four aspects of experience to which you can pay attention: the body, sensations, emotions and thoughts, and context and perspective.[17]

The Body

First you become aware of the body in all its aspects as you sit, stand, walk, or lie down. As you'll see in part 3 of this book, this doesn't mean looking at the body from the outside in a detached way but in a manner that's integrated, embodied, and alive; it means truly *inhabiting* the body.

Sensations

Second, you become aware of sensations and your responses to them. You continually perceive sensations—the eyes see, the ears hear, the nose smells, the tongue tastes, and the body touches—and you notice whether you find these pleasant, unpleasant, or somewhere in between. You also perceive thoughts, memories, and fantasies, and find these pleasant or unpleasant. Usually we react to pleasant sensations by wanting to have more of them and to unpleasant ones by wishing them away. But mindfully noticing experience means seeing what it actually is, rather than being locked into distorted thinking based on craving and aversion. Then you can find the moment in which choice is possible before your habitual reactions take over. For those of us living with physical pain or illness, it's vital to recognize that our pain is *just* pain; then you can interrupt the layers of resistance and aversion that create your secondary suffering instead of being a victim of your impulses.

Emotions and Thoughts

Most of us identify so strongly with our emotions and thoughts that we feel that we *are* them. But mindfulness means seeing thoughts more objectively. For example, if my pain worsens, I can imagine a host of terrible consequences stretching into the future. But these thoughts are probably just expressions of my anxiety. If I can see that they're just thoughts, rather than "buying in" to them, I'll be better able to see what's really happening and respond constructively. In this way you see that emotions and thoughts aren't fixed or solid facts, but are always changing. This helps you to take more responsibility for your state of mind. When you feel angry or upset it's easy to blame others, but it's your own anger, and you can choose to prolong it or to calm down. There's more on this in the section on working with thoughts in chapter 16.

Context and Perspective

Finally, there's your perspective on your experience.[18] With time, mindfulness practice can open the door to a profound shift in your whole outlook on life, and a wise, deep perspective on your experience can emerge. This points to the next dimension of mindfulness.

The Nature of What I'm Aware Of

Usually we experience things as if they're fixed and unchanging. We say, "That's just the way I am," and we see others in the same way: "I don't like her because she's an angry person," "He's so grumpy," and so on. But mindfulness helps us notice that everything changes continually. We change from moment to moment as different thoughts, feelings, and sensations come into our experience, and other people continually change, too. The world around us is also more fluid than we think: night turns to day; summer becomes winter; mountains erode. Nothing is exempt from this law, and when you really take this in you are able to relax into the flow of change. A Buddhist text says:

> *Thus shall you think of all in this fleeting world:*
> *A star at dawn, a bubble in a stream;*
> *A flash of lightning in a summer cloud,*
> *A flickering lamp, a phantom, and a dream.*[19]

This shift in perspective can be particularly striking for those of us living with pain if we use mindfulness practice to investigate the actual nature of the pain in this moment. You can gradually tease apart the different aspects of an experience — the basic physical sensations, the resistance that arises in your mind and body, emotions such as grief and anger, and thoughts connected with the pain. You may also discover that your experience includes elements that are pleasant.

Such investigation shows that pain is a constantly shifting *process*, and it's bound up with your responses to it. Pain certainly is unpleasant; that's its nature, but if you explore the sensations in your body and let go of your ideas about them, your memories of the past, and your fears about the future, they can even become fascinating. It's hard to engage with pain like this, but you'll suffer less because you're dropping the burden of secondary suffering that arises when you perceive your pain as fixed and unchanging and then react to it.

It's the same with states of mind. Depression, fatigue, anger, happiness, and joy are labels for processes that are continually changing. Seeing how anger, for example, arises and passes away can make it easier to let go of it and make creative choices.[20]

COMMON HUMANITY AND EMPATHY

Mindfulness practice also includes awareness of other people. The aspects of mindfulness I've mentioned so far — inhabiting your body moment by moment and knowing your sensations, emotions, and thoughts — all foster self-awareness. From this basis you can broaden your awareness and imaginatively identify with other people's experience. We all have a body that experiences sensations, we all have thoughts and emotions, and we all try to avoid pain and cling to pleasure in broadly similar ways.

The Buddhist writer Jeffrey Hopkins describes traveling with the Dalai Lama on his first visit to the West.[21] Wherever he went, the Dalai Lama repeated one main message: "Everybody wants to be happy; nobody wants to suffer." Hopkins had heard the Dalai Lama give long philosophical teachings and wondered why he was making such a simple point. Then he realized how different his own experience would be if he really internalized the truth that behind our different personalities and actions lies the same basic desire to avoid suffering and to be happy. If he related to others on the basis of that common humanity, his experience would be transformed from one of isolation to one of empathy.

TURNING PAIN UPSIDE DOWN AND INSIDE OUT

This is a vital shift for those of us living with chronic illness and pain. The very pain that tends to isolate us can become a source of connection if we can see that, one way or another, at one time or another, everybody experiences pain. This radical shift in perspective turns pain inside out and upside down. If you accept pain and explore it more deeply, instead of ruining your life, it can open you to life — it's just your own particular version of the human predicament. Opening to your own pain means that you know by imaginative identification what it's like for others to suffer. Cultivating an attitude of kindness and care toward yourself creates a foundation from which you can extend kindness to others. This is the principle behind the kindly awareness practice, which is at the heart of my approach to mindfulness and will be described fully in chapter 15.

When I talk about this in Breathworks courses, I see lightbulbs going off in people's minds. Participants often assume initially that others on the course are fine (because pain is an invisible condition for many), but as they hear each other's stories they realize that difficulty is universal; this helps them to relate to others as rounded human beings rather than as expressions of all the things they lack. I sometimes do an exercise in which people sit quietly in threes, and each has a minute or so to name the unpleasant aspects of his or her immediate experience: "Cold feet — unpleasant. Tightness in stomach — unpleasant. Pain in left shoulder — unpleasant." Then we repeat the exercise with each person naming pleasant sensations: "Warm hands — pleasant. Tingling in left earlobe — pleasant. Softness in face — pleasant." Following this, we sit in silence with a sense of all we have in common. I like listening to the murmuring in the room as people name their experience. It's a striking way of seeing that everyone's life includes unpleasant and pleasant elements and that our experiences are, in essence, similar.

> ✳ **JOHN**
>
> The biggest thing for John about being in a Breathworks course was recognizing that his pain didn't isolate him; in fact, it was his pain that made him human. He saw that everybody experiences pain to some degree, and it isn't unique to him. Instead of feeling isolated and apart, he can use it as a way of engaging with other people.

One time, when my back pain was particularly awful, I lay in bed and dropped into the pain, and with each breath I softened my resistance to it. I felt I was dropping so far into my body and my life that I fell out of the bottom of "me." I sensed a powerful connection with all the other people who were suffering in that moment: children in African villages, women in childbirth, people who were dying. I didn't find connectedness by looking out of myself but by engaging so deeply with my experience of pain that I emerged into something much stiller. The thought came to me: *I'm not special. This is not a special experience. This is something that many people are having right now, and I can feel for those people because of what I'm experiencing.* Instead of thinking, *Why me, why am I the one with so much pain?* the question became, *Why not me? Why should I not experience pain when it's part of the human condition?* I don't think I could have felt that level of empathy without the pain I was experiencing. As the poet Rilke said:

> *The doves that remained at home, never exposed to loss,*
> *Innocent and secure, cannot know tenderness;*
> *Only the won-back heart can ever be satisfied: free,*
> *through all it has given up, to rejoice in its mastery.*[22]

❋ **SARA**

Sara liked the unpleasant/pleasant awareness exercise we did in class. At one point she could hear different voices naming their pain, and she had a sense of the courage in the room. She went from feeling down before she started the class to lying on the floor at home in the evening, listening to music and playing with her cat. She had the same amount of pain, but having connected with others she felt utterly content.

AWARENESS AND KINDNESS

Mindfulness in its fullness is imbued with kindness. In the Buddhist tradition it is said that wisdom and compassion are like two wings of a bird, and mindfulness can help us cultivate both.

Wisdom comes from having a more accurate perception of life. It's wise to let go of the ideas, stories, and reactions that overlie experience; it's also wise to see more deeply into the fluid and changing nature of both painful and pleasurable experience as if it were coming into being and passing away like waves on the ocean.

Kindness and compassion arise when we extend that perception to other people. It's moving to see how human beings face the same difficulties and are propelled by the same tendencies. We live them out uniquely, but we enact the same dramas and struggle with the same predicaments.

INTERCONNECTEDNESS AND KINDNESS

The truth is that we aren't separate and isolated from one another. Whenever we speak or act, we affect others, and this influences the way they themselves behave. If I get angry with people at work, they may take their frustration out on their kids when they get home, and the kids, in turn, may respond by getting into trouble. On the other hand, being kind will lead to different consequences. You never know how far the ripples reach.

THE NET OF JEWELS

Imagine a vast net that stretches in all directions of space. A single glittering jewel hangs at each link of the net, and since the net itself is infinite in all dimensions, the jewels are infinite in number. If you look closely at any one of these jewels, you see that its polished surface reflects all the other jewels in the net. Life is like this, and each of us is like a jewel in this image—continually affecting, and being affected by, all the other jewels.[23]

CHAPTER 5

The Five-Step Model of Mindfulness

Inside this new love . . .
Become the sky . . .
Escape . . .
Walk out like someone suddenly born into color.
Do it now.
You're covered with thick cloud.
Slide out the side . . .
Your old life was a frantic running
from silence.
The speechless full moon
comes out now.

RUMI[1]

Now that you have a sense of the dimensions of mindfulness, it's time to explore how to develop it, as mindfulness is a way of living that's cultivated by practice. Few people live with continual awareness, so for most of us mindfulness training means becoming aware once you're already distracted. You'll probably find yourself caught up in distractions hundreds of times a day, but choosing awareness even once is a victory, no matter how fleeting that moment may be. It's a step in retraining yourself after years of unhelpful habitual behavior. In time, awareness itself becomes a habit.

Mindfulness practice is like any other training. If you want to become an athlete, you need to develop certain muscles so you can run with ease; to cultivate mindfulness you must train your awareness so that it becomes an increasingly reliable source of strength and stability. This chapter describes five steps or progressive stages in developing mindfulness that offer a realistic and sustainable approach to practice for those of us living with pain and illness. I have included a short mindfulness exercise with the first four steps. (You can find an audio version of the exercises at soundstrue.com/burch.)

STEP ONE
THE STARTING POINT: AWARENESS

The first step in developing mindfulness is simply to become more familiar with what's actually happening in each moment. For example, you can become aware of your breath; of your body as you sit, walk, stand, or lie down; and of your sensations — pleasant or painful. You can notice your thoughts and emotions as discrete aspects of your experience instead of overidentifying with them. You can become more aware of other people and the world around you. You might suddenly notice little things such as the sensation of the sun on your skin, the taste of an orange, or the greenness of the grass on a summer's day. Becoming more aware can be like moving from a two-dimensional, black-and-white world to one that has three dimensions and is saturated with color.

> **EXERCISE: PRESENT-MOMENT AWARENESS**
>
> Notice what you're experiencing right now. Can you feel the book in your hands as you hold it? Is it warm or cold, rough or soft, heavy or light? Does holding it feel comfortable? Are your shoulders relaxed or hunched? What about your belly: is it tight or soft? What happens when you bring your attention to these areas? Do they relax a little? Feel free to shift your posture in any way you want as you become more aware.

Now notice the sensations of contact between your body and your support. Does your body feel heavy or light, relaxed or tense? Just notice how your body feels without judging your experience.

How does the breath in your body feel in this moment? What parts of your body move with the breath?

What sounds and smells are you aware of?

How many colors can you see? Can you simply enjoy them, noticing all the different shades and textures?

As you draw this exercise to a close, see if you can carry this quality of awareness into the rest of your day, being alert, engaged, and curious about your experience.

STEP TWO
MOVE TOWARD THE UNPLEASANT

The second step — moving toward unpleasant aspects of experience — is deeply counterintuitive and probably comes as a surprise. It may even sound masochistic. In fact, facing pain is essential because those of us with chronic pain usually resist it through trying to block the pain out or else drowning in it. In neither case do we really see the pain for what it is.

When you first turn your attention to painful sensations, you may be more aware of your resistance than of the pain itself, but you can work with this by gently "leaning into" the resistance with your awareness and using your breath to drop your awareness more deeply into your body. You can breathe in with a sense of awareness and breathe out with a sense of letting go.

Over time you can learn to adopt a kindly, nonjudgmental attitude to the whole of your experience and allow painful sensations simply to be present. You can develop a caring attitude toward your pain — like that of the natural impulse of a mother to gather a child who is hurt into her arms and hold him or her tenderly. Even though she can't remove the child's pain, her loving response will ease his or her distress.

❋ REBECCA

Rebecca has been disabled since birth and has been through more than forty operations. She has meditated for many years and recently told me how turning toward the pain has helped her:

Turning toward the pain meant facing the fear that it would get out of control and I'd be overwhelmed. I'd never really looked into the pain, and that meant I'd turned it into a monster. So I tried to look at the monster. What shape was it? Where exactly was it located? Did it have a color? I became interested in the pain's real nature. I found that however bad it was, it didn't kill me! I discovered that some kinds of pain are more bearable than others; for instance, I can bear more of a fresh pain than old, nagging pain. I also saw how I solidify the idea of pain, as if it were a hot and jagged mountain. But when I turn toward it I see that it changes from moment to moment, and noticing those differences helped me to experience the pain instead of being caught in reactions.

Taking Things One Moment at a Time

It's easy to think that moving toward the pain will add to the sense of drowning, as Rebecca feared. But feeling overwhelmed usually comes from being overidentified with ideas about experience. You think, *Oh my God, this is awful. I can't bear it. I hate my life. I've had this pain for ten years and it will never go away. It's getting worse; I feel so tired. I won't be able to go out with my friends and they'll reject me. No wonder I have no friends left.* Before you know it, you're caught up in thoughts about how your pain stretches interminably into the past and will continue indefinitely into the future.

When you bring awareness and curiosity to the actual *experience* of pain, often you find that it's not as bad as you feared. Focusing on direct perception of the sensations rather than ideas about them brings you into the present moment in which experience is always fluid and changing. You see that you only ever experience your pain one moment at a time — as I understood in the hospital experience I described in chapter 1 (see page 5). The fear that I couldn't get through until morning dissolved when I realized that I simply had to live each moment, that the present moment is always bearable, and that the only authentic and sustainable way to be fully alive is to be open to all life's moments, not just the ones I prefer.

EXERCISE: MOVING TOWARD THE UNPLEASANT

As you sit or lie down, gently open your awareness to include any unpleasant or painful sensations. Let them enter your field of awareness with an attitude of tenderness and kindly curiosity. Remember to keep breathing! We commonly tense against pain and hold the breath, but see if you can soften *toward* the pain with gentle breaths.

Maybe you are more aware of a sense of resistance and tension than of the pain itself. If so, see if you can investigate this resistance a little more directly—turning your attention toward it, like shining a soft light onto something that's hidden in shadow. Maybe you can "lean into" it with your awareness, as if you were gently leaning against a dense, yet pliant, object. Allow it to soften a little with each in- and out-breath. Maybe you can feel the resistance softening as you let the body settle onto the earth with each out-breath.

As you open to the pain itself, notice what the actual sensations are like and sense how they are always changing. Maybe they feel hard and tight one moment, a little softer the next? Or are they sharp one moment and then tingly?

Can you tell exactly where the pain is located in your body? Be precise about this. You may notice that the pain is more localized than you thought.

This may be the first time you've investigated your pain directly, so be patient with any disturbed thoughts or feelings of fear and anxiety that may arise. Notice how these are also constantly changing. See if you can relax a little around whatever unpleasant experiences you notice, and remember to let the weight of your body settle down onto the earth beneath you and soften your breath each time you notice you're tensing.

STEP THREE
SEEKING THE PLEASANT

This third step in developing mindfulness in fact grows naturally out of the second, but it may seem even more surprising: it involves becoming sensitive to the *pleasant* elements of your experience. Hardening against pain also shuts out the pleasurable side of life, and we lose the sensitivity that allows us to feel vibrantly alive and experience pleasure and love. You might not feel the pain so much, but you'll numb yourself to other people, the beauty of nature, or the simple pleasure of the body's warmth while sitting in the sun. When I've been most able to be with my pain as a changing, dynamic experience, I've also been most in touch with the poignancy and subtlety of the human condition and most able to appreciate the world around me.

As you develop a more straightforward relationship with pain, you make the surprising discovery that there's always something pleasant, even beautiful, in your experience when you look for it. Everyone I've worked with, even those suffering severe pain, has found something pleasant to focus on, and for those of us living with chronic pain or illness this can be a revelation.

Seeking the pleasant is like being an explorer searching for hidden treasure. It might be as simple as noting the warmth of your hands or a pleasant feeling in the belly, or seeing a shaft of sunlight streaming through the window. If you're in the hospital it could be the smell of flowers by your bed or the pleasure of being with someone you love: maybe you notice the way their eyes crinkle when they smile or the quality of their touch as they hold your hand.

As I've become more mindful, I'm much more attuned to the subtleties of my sensations. I notice how my hair feels against my forehead; when I meditate with my eyes closed, I notice the contact between my eyes and eyelids. Through such sensitivity the present moment becomes richer, more multifaceted, and more alive.

What to Do If You Can't Find Anything Pleasant

If you have a lot of pain the suggestion that there is something pleasurable in your experience may seem laughable. You'll need to explore this area with an open mind and a willingness to experience new things, letting go of any fixed ideas about your experience. You may be surprised.

A few years ago I was in the hospital following surgery, having developed an infection that caused tremendous pain. As I searched for pleasant sensations, I noticed I was enjoying the contact between my body and the crisp, clean bedsheets. That moment was particularly beautiful because the contrast with the pain made the feeling more pleasurable than usual.

Seeking the Pleasant Isn't Simply Distraction

Well-meaning friends and professionals may have encouraged you to "think positively" when you're in pain. That can be good advice, but you may simply be painting a veneer of false positivity over your suffering, which is just another form of avoidance. Seeking out pleasant aspects of experience as the third step of mindfulness is different. In the second step you have acknowledged your pain with kindness, rather than trying to distract yourself from it or blocking it out. This attitude of sensitivity, openness, and honesty to the whole of your experience, including your pain, now allows you to gently turn to the pleasant aspects of the moment that have been there all along, just outside your field of awareness. You can feel stable and whole, rather than grasping for pleasure to avoid your pain. Amazing as it can seem, pleasure is always present, but you close yourself to it when dominated by your pain. As you let in pleasurable sensations, you may feel relief that you're at last giving them attention.

EXERCISE: SEEKING THE PLEASANT

Start off by being aware of your whole body as you sit or lie down. Notice the breath rising and falling, and allow your body to rest down toward the earth, particularly on each out-breath.

If pain is present, let go of any tendency to tense up, and gently shift your focus to notice anything that's pleasant in this moment—like focusing the close-up lens of a camera on a beautiful object.

Notice pleasant physical sensations first of all, no matter how subtle they may be. It might be a sense of warmth in your hands, a pleasant tingling somewhere in your body, or perhaps a sense of relief around the heart area now that you're allowing yourself to come to rest with your experience in its wholeness. Maybe there's a curious sensation in your left earlobe that you realize is pleasant! Spend some time moving through your body with your awareness and pause when you find something pleasurable.

Now expand your awareness and notice any pleasant sounds. Spend a few moments simply appreciating them as sounds. Notice any tendency to get caught up in wondering about their source or wanting them to last. Just let them rise and fall.

Look around you and notice anything that's beautiful or pleasant in your immediate environment. It might be the light in the room or a picture on the wall. Just appreciate it as if you're seeing it for the first time.

❋ **DEBBIE**

Debbie lives with severe musculoskeletal pain and fatigue, and she came to the Breathworks course when she was down and exhausted. She laughed out loud when she heard about looking for pleasant aspects of her experience. It seemed ludicrous that she might feel anything but unremitting pain and despair. But as she sat preparing to meditate, she noticed the wall in front of her and realized she was appreciating the care that had gone into the brickwork. It was a revelation to find that often there were pleasant things in her experience that she usually didn't notice because she was so identified with her pain.

STEP FOUR
BROADENING AWARENESS TO BECOME A BIGGER CONTAINER AND CULTIVATING EQUANIMITY

In the fourth step you broaden your awareness to include both the unpleasant and pleasant aspects of your experience, like switching from a focused to a wide-angle lens. In this stage, rather than focusing closely on sensations of pain or pleasure, you become aware of the diverse aspects of each moment as they come into being and pass away without automatically pushing away the unpleasant or clinging to the pleasant. Practicing mindfulness isn't about escaping difficulty; it's about holding the whole of experience in a wider perspective with equanimity and depth.

The Zen teacher Charlotte Joko Beck calls this state "becoming a bigger container."[2] Often you feel too small to accommodate what happens, as if you are a restrictive and narrow container. That causes stress. But if you feel yourself to be a bigger container, you can manage whatever happens and maintain perspective with a deep sense of inner spaciousness. Ultimately, the container may be limitless and allow a sense of space, freedom, and stability.

If you put a teaspoon of salt in a small glass of water it will have a strong taste, but if you add the same amount of salt to a lake, the water will be largely unaffected. With mindfulness you can become like a deep and clear lake: individual experiences don't overwhelm you, and you can remain steady through life's ups and downs while being honest about what's happening.

It can be a huge relief to accept the whole of your experience. It allows you to relax much more deeply. When you experience the sensations of your body right here, right now, whatever they may be, you can rest within it, settling your awareness in the stability of the belly rather than identifying with anxious thoughts in your head about your pain or illness. Truly settling in the body feels like coming home.

A Sense of Connectedness with Others

Another aspect of this fourth step is to become sensitive to and aware of other people. You may notice how you communicate with your friends and family and how they communicate with you. As you feel greater emotional robustness and become more able to take things in, you may become less touchy and shrug off difficulties rather than being dragged down by them. You can relax and enjoy other people's company much more.

EXERCISE: OPENING TO THE WHOLE OF EXPERIENCE

Bring your awareness to your whole experience as you sit or lie down reading this book. Notice the contact between your hands and the book and the broader sense of your body on the chair or the bed. Gather your awareness around the breath for a few moments. See if you can feel from the inside how the breath gently rocks the body, and settle down onto the earth with each breath. You might imagine you're floating on a gentle ocean swell being rocked by the constant, rhythmic movement.

Imagine all the different aspects of your experience in this moment are taking place within a broad and open field of awareness. Let everything rise and fall with a fluid sense of change and flow, neither pushing away painful experience nor clinging to things you find pleasant. You'll probably find you relax for a moment and then get caught up in particular experiences. Never mind. Every time you notice a moment of resistance or clinging you can relax back down again into a sense of breadth and openness. Allow your awareness to be centered down in your belly.

Let your awareness be open and inclusive, including everything, whether it's an internal experience or something you perceive through your senses, such as a sound.

Awareness of the World

A final dimension of the bigger container is becoming aware of the world around you. I had a strong experience of this in my late twenties when I spent eighteen months making a film based on images from nature. Meditation was teaching me to "be," and that enabled me to become aware of the world around me instead of running away from my pain. I could no longer climb and hike, but photography allowed me to combine my love of nature with my pleasure in making things. The film was stimulated by my hospital experience and my curiosity about time and space and the mystery of the timeless present moment.

As I traveled through some of the most beautiful places in New Zealand, I was trying to see more deeply into the world. I would lie on my back looking up at the sky—blue as only New Zealand skies can be—and photograph the endlessly changing clouds and colors. I photographed black iron sand on a volcanic beach so close up that it could have been an image of a galaxy: flames leaping and dancing, shattering the illusion that a frozen image might halt the fire's relentless movement; smooth water fracturing into the hectic cascades of a rapid. I learned to see the incredible beauty in the depths of things and the constantly changing nature of matter and how it's impossible to hang on to anything because the nature of everything is change. How can you grasp a handful of clouds? As soon as I captured an image of a wave, it was gone.

My quest was to appreciate life's exquisite beauty without clinging to it with a grasping fist, to be open to the textures of the world around me while allowing experience to slip through open fingers. These fascinations have stayed with me ever since, and they hold important lessons for my own life.

STEP FIVE

CHOICE: LEARNING TO RESPOND, RATHER THAN REACT

With this wider perspective you can move on to the fifth step: choosing to *respond* rather than *react* to your experiences, especially when they include difficulties.[3] The sense that you have the freedom to choose how you respond is the heart of mindfulness practice.

In a sense, each of the five steps involves choice: you choose to start noticing your experience rather than avoiding it, to move *toward the painful* and *seek out the pleasant* aspects, and to broaden out your awareness. These stages tease apart the different aspects of experience, helping you distinguish between primary suffering — the actual painful or unpleasant sensations — and secondary suffering, which springs from your resistance to them. This creates a sense of spaciousness, as if you're a bigger container. Rather than feeling your pain is right on top of you and you're trapped in a battle that leaves no space to choose your response, you can find ways to respond creatively to any circumstances with a soft and pliant heart. The previous steps of mindfulness prepare the way for you to act with initiative and confidence.

When life is approached in this way, with mindfulness, it can be a stream of choices and creative possibilities instead of continuous distraction and resistance.

Here's an example from my diary of how I work with this myself:

Today I woke up feeling tired and nauseous but also willing myself to do my writing as I'd planned. I wanted to override the back pain, fatigue, and nausea. I felt myself hardening against my pain, and the

*tension grew in my body. Then I caught myself and decided I would
stop, lie down, and listen to a meditation CD. By the end I felt that
I'd broken out of an old groove of behavior and I had more perspective.
I realized it didn't really matter whether I got my writing finished
today. Now it's 5:30 and the writing is flowing. I'm using my timer
to remind me to take a break after twenty minutes at my desk, and
when I hear it beeping I again face the choice: do I react by ignoring
it, or do I respond by lying down?*

Mindfulness Is Not Suppression

It's easy to hear about the value of responding, not reacting, and to
think that you shouldn't react. You might judge difficult emotions and
think that you've failed in mindfulness practice if you feel moody or
irritable. But mindfulness is being *honestly* aware of what's happening,
not pasting on a layer of false equanimity. If you feel grumpy, the
practice is to be aware of that without judging, and then you can find
the best way to respond.

Living with pain is hard, so it's understandable if you feel emotions
such as grumpiness or anger, but if you can acknowledge those
feelings when they arise, then you will find space around them. Such
emotions often feed on themselves in an escalating spiral of blame,
self-pity, and rage, but it's always possible to find moments in which
you can choose to encourage more helpful states of mind. It isn't easy,
and it may be humiliating to face your negativity, but each time you
manage this, it's a little taste of freedom.

One of the main emotional effects of my pain is that I can get
impatient and grumpy, especially in lengthy discussions or group
situations that require patience. If there's a decision to be made, I just
want to make it quickly, and behind this is the thought that the sooner
I finish, the sooner I'll be able to lie down. But this attitude is hard for
others, and it has affected my relationships and friendships. I wish it
wasn't like this, but I'm finding that the best thing is just to own up to

feeling irritable when it happens instead of thinking I can prevent it ever arising. My mindfulness practice helps me to notice what's happening without being too defensive and to take steps to behave differently.

Recently I was on a training retreat, and my colleague Ratnaguna demonstrated this honest and authentic aspect of mindfulness very well. When we had a meeting to discuss the retreat program he seemed withdrawn, and before long he told me that he felt irritable. But he communicated this without blaming anyone. His meditation experience meant he could be precise and uncomplicated in evaluating what he was feeling, so it was easy to empathize with him. He also knew from past experience that this kind of irritability grows out of sadness; he simply needed time alone to be with his experience, and he knew that it would then settle and pass. I found it inspiring that Ratnaguna could be honest about his difficult emotions without suppressing them or overidentifying with them and that he had the courage to move toward the sadness underlying them, giving it the space to subside naturally.

SPECIAL ISSUES FOR PRACTICING MINDFULNESS WITH PAIN AND ILLNESS

Mindfulness can sound deceptively simple, so I want to go into a few more areas that are particularly relevant to those of us living with pain or illness.

Working with Intense Pain

Sometimes the experience of physical pain is so intense that you just can't work with it using awareness, no matter how much meditation, relaxation, or other techniques you've practiced. It's important not to feel you've failed if you're overwhelmed by your physical experience; it's still possible to get back on track.

After my last surgery I was in the hospital for six weeks. Until the last few days I felt emotionally positive and managed to maintain equanimity and patience, but then the pain grew very intense, and I fell into fear, despondency, and self-pity. A friend visited and I moaned about another friend by whom I felt let down. When she left I felt even worse: not only did I have to cope with my pain, I also felt guilty about my reaction and its effect on my friend. The next morning I phoned her and apologized; I immediately felt better. I began the slow climb out of the pit and learned an important lesson: even when I was in the most hellish state and couldn't stop my reactions, I could still rectify the situation later by finding a moment of choice.

Prescription Medication and Mindfulness

People sometimes think they can't practice mindfulness and take painkillers, tranquilizers, antidepressants, and so on, as they affect the mind. In my view there's no inherent conflict. Some drugs do cloud the mind, but severe pain clouds it as well. If I reduce my medication too far, I end up tense and exhausted, which doesn't help me develop awareness, so I take several pain medications at a dose worked out with my pain-management consultant. The key is to find an optimum dose that leaves the mind as clear as possible without becoming overwhelmed by the pain.

Practicing mindfulness does help many people to feel more relaxed and happy—and also to sleep better, allowing them to reduce medication such as tranquilizers or sleeping pills. Keep in mind that you should always make adjustments to your medication in consultation with a health professional.

Distraction and Mindfulness

Does developing mindfulness of experience, including pain, mean there's no place for distraction? I think it has a place if you take into account your motivation and whether your condition is acute or chronic. With acute pain that you know will pass, it can help to take your mind off it to do something more enjoyable than simply watching the pain. But with a chronic condition, continually distracting yourself may create a habit of avoidance that, in fact, brings greater suffering. If a mother ignores a crying child because she's busy, the child will just cry louder, and the mother's activity becomes more stressful because of the background screaming. But if the child is given some attention he or she may calm down, and then the mother can relax as well. A painful body is similar. If you include the pain in your awareness, you can accommodate it within a broad perspective while getting on with other things and pursuing your interests. This approach makes for a more fulfilling and successful life in the long run.

I call the attempt to escape and deny painful experience "compulsive distraction," but an alternative is "aware diversion," when you consciously choose to take your mind off the pain by engaging with something else. There's definitely a place for this within mindfulness-based pain management. Often I decide to read a novel or watch a movie as a stimulating and enjoyable way to relax and have downtime. Choosing consciously to do so feels very different from just rushing from one distraction to another.

CHAPTER 6

Healing: Becoming Whole

Ah, not to be cut off,
not through the slightest partition
shut out from the law of the stars.
The inner — what is it?
If not intensified sky,
hurled through with birds and deep
with the winds of homecoming.

RAINER MARIA RILKE[1]

In modern medicine the emphasis on finding a cure for whatever is affecting your health is wonderful if your condition can be cured, but it's less well equipped to deal with incurable conditions that bring chronic pain and illness. When Christopher Reeve, the actor who played Superman, was paralyzed from the neck down in a riding accident, he used his celebrity to promote research into curing spinal-cord injuries (SCI), and he became a leading figure in this search. Until his death in 2005, he worked tirelessly at his rehab so that his muscles would remain in good condition for when science had found a cure for paralysis. His efforts led to major developments in the understanding of SCI, but the publicity surrounding the new research also encouraged some newly injured people to believe that a cure was just around the corner; they saw no point in becoming proficient wheelchair users and didn't work at their rehab. Passively waiting for a cure meant that their lives were, in fact, more diminished than they would have been had they learned to make the best of the situation by adapting to an active life in a wheelchair.

Of course it's important that researchers do all they can to develop scientific understanding and make new treatments available. But those of us with chronic conditions also need strategies to help us live well in the here and now, and many people in medicine and psychology who work in pain management recognize the importance of acceptance in learning to live with pain. Mindfulness can play a vital role in this process. While it might not cure your condition, it can be part of a profound process of healing.

Mindfulness and healing are both concerned with becoming more integrated and whole. Even if you can't be whole physically because of damage, surgery, or disease, you can still experience a healthy and whole relationship between your body and your mind, between yourself and the world. These connections can even be sacred: the words *healing, health, holy,* and *wholeness* all come from the same etymological root.[2] Wholeness in this sense is the real key to happiness and inner peace.

Integration is another word connected with wholeness and comes from the Latin *integratio,* which means "renewal" or "restoration to wholeness." In my experience, moments of mindful wholeness feel like a homecoming, in which something that I intuitively recognize as healthy and true is restored. When I'm fragmented, fractured, and scattered, I also know that I'm in some sense exiled and cut off from "the intensified sky" of the inner world that Rilke mentions. Mindfulness practice is a journey to wholeness.

THE DISTINCTION BETWEEN HEALING AND CURE

It's important not to confuse this deep healing with simple ideas of "cure." I can't mend my spine with the power of my mind or restore the paralyzed nerves, but I *can* change my relationship with my condition and find peace in my body. Jon Kabat-Zinn describes his work at the

Center for Mindfulness at the University of Massachusetts Medical School as "healing," even though many participants in his courses have conditions that mainstream medicine considers untreatable:

> What we mean above all is that the course participants are undergoing a profound transformation of view. This transformation is brought about by the encounter with one's own wholeness, catalyzed by the meditation practice. When we glimpse our own completeness in the stillness of any moment . . . a new and profound coming to terms with our problems and our suffering begins to take place. We begin to see both ourselves and our problems differently, namely from the perspective of wholeness. This transformation of view creates an entirely different context within which we can see and work with our problems, however serious they may be. It's a perceptual shift away from fragmentation and isolation toward wholeness and connectedness. With this change of perspective comes a shift from feeling out of control and beyond help (helpless and pessimistic) to a sense of the possible, a sense of acceptance, and inner peace and control.[3]

Those who learn mindfulness while living with terminal illness confront the distinction between healing and cure most starkly of all. We'll all face death one day, so death is a part of everyone's life, but as Stephen Levine suggested in his book *Healing into Life and Death*, even if you are dying, you can still heal yourself by changing your relationship with your experience.[4] In this sense healing doesn't mean the absence of symptoms, disease, or disability, and you only discover what it really means by embarking on your own, very personal healing journey. That journey, which often includes coming to terms with your situation and letting go of an unrealistic search for a cure, is often long and complex. It takes time to see the need to heal your *attitude* to your difficulties.

MY PATH TO WHOLENESS

Looking back on more than thirty years since I first injured my back in 1976, I see that I've been through a healing journey with three distinct phases of about ten years (which are similar to the stages of grieving outlined by Elisabeth Kübler-Ross).[5] While the details of my experience are unique, these phases seem to be what human beings commonly go through when faced with the impossible problem: how do I accept the unacceptable?

Phase One: Denial

For the ten years following the onset of my condition, I ignored my pain and attempted to live a normal life. In fact, I tried to be even more active than others. I cycled and swam frenetically to prove that I still could; I worked sixty hours a week, sometimes continuing through the night to meet deadlines. If anyone asked me about my pain I blushed and had to leave the room, and I secretly took painkillers in the bathroom at work.

Pain was my enemy, and I willed myself, through sheer effort and determination, to exist in a sort of pain-free parallel universe. I didn't even acknowledge my pain and distress to myself; I was furious with my body for its frailty and for having betrayed me, and when bullying it didn't work, I exiled it into unawareness. When I think about that young woman now, I feel such sadness that she didn't know any other way to be.

Phase Two: Bargaining

Ten years after my original injury and two years after the car crash, my denial ran out, and I hit a wall of exhaustion. I had the major crisis described at the beginning of this book, and I could no longer ignore my body. For the first time I stepped onto the path of aware-ness. I left my career in film, started to meditate, and tried to take responsibility for myself. I practiced yoga (vigorously, of course!), visited complementary therapists, and began the slow and painful process of reengaging with my body. This was frightening and overwhelming, but I had started the journey home.

In this phase, which lasted another ten years, I engaged in helpful practices, but I did so as part of an implicit bargain. My motivation was to make my difficulties go away: *If I do yoga I can cure my back. Osteopathy will cure me. Meditation will make my pain end.* These treatments did help and I experienced more peace of mind, but my experience was still strained because deep down I thought the only way I could be healed was if my condition was cured. Periodically the pain came crashing back with terrible brutality. When that happened, I felt as if I'd failed and that I needed to try even harder, only to become even more confused and despondent when the pain persisted. And so the cycle continued, leaving me emotionally barren and desperate. I knew I was doing all the right things, but I still wasn't achieving the results I longed for.

Phase Three: Acceptance

In 1997 another crisis came when my condition deteriorated, paralyzing my bowel and bladder and partially paralyzing my legs. I started to use a wheelchair and needed major surgery to reconstruct my lower spine. This was another difficult time, and I had to go deep within myself to acknowledge that I had harmed myself through my bargaining attitude and lack of acceptance. I was paying the price for recklessly pushing my body.

In the five years between my relapse and the surgery that improved things in 2002, I spent more months flat on my back and still more years largely housebound. It was a dark voyage. In addition to my pain, I had to face my deepest and most destructive habits, especially my tendency to overdo things and then "crash and burn." I slowly rehabilitated myself and built up my strength again, but this time I did so on a more kindly and realistic basis, and I practiced mindfulness of daily activities with a new commitment.

During this time I began to formulate the Breathworks program. I'd learned a lot — as much from my mistakes as from my victories. Running the courses took me out of myself and broadened my horizons. The spirit I saw rising up again and again in others in the most difficult circumstances played a big part in my own rehabilitation.

Imperceptibly, I've entered a third phase of healing: acceptance. Sometimes people confuse acceptance with resignation and passivity, but the Latin root of acceptance is *capere*, which means "to take." Acceptance means actively taking hold of experience in a realistic and conscious way. I practice the same methods — meditation, swimming, osteopathy, massage, and so on — but I do so with a more peaceful attitude. I'm motivated to maintain what function and mobility I have, but my underlying quest is no longer to get rid of or overcome my pain. It's simply to abide in my body as it is and to be as alive and awake as possible in each moment. I accept that my body is damaged in ways that cannot be undone and that pain will be my constant companion. I don't like it, but I'm not fighting it as I used to, and it no longer dominates my life.

Recently I read a remarkable memoir by Matthew Sandford, who became paralyzed from the chest down at the age of thirteen in a terrible car accident that killed both his father and sister. For twenty-eight years he has been on a similar journey to my own, and he's now a yoga teacher. For many years Matthew tried to overcome his difficulties using willpower, and he experienced a schism between his mind and his body:

> *Imagine walking from a well-lit room into a dark one. Imagine the darkness as a visual expression of silence (caused by disowning the body). My rehabilitation . . . taught me to willfully strike out against the darkness. It told me to move faster rather than slower, push*

*harder rather than softer. It guided me to compensate for what I could
not see. My arms and my [wheelchair], fueled by a compensating
will, were to carry me through my life. My efforts would aim to prove
that the room's darkness didn't matter at all. I would overcome it and
become as effective as if the light was still on.*[6]

I recognize that dark room from my own years of denial and bargaining and the effort to fight it. Matthew's turning point came when he asked what would happen if he could "work with the darkness."[7] Rather than overcoming it, this meant being patient:

*Stop moving, wait for the eyes to adjust, allow for stillness, and
then see what's possible. Although full-fledged vision does not
return, usually there is enough light to find one's way across the
room. After a while, the moon may come out, sounds might gain
texture, and the world might reveal itself once again, only darker.*[8]

In his twenties, Matthew discovered yoga and started to pay attention to the subtlest level of his physical experience. Through this, he found that the relationship of the mind to the body is truly mysterious:

*If I listen inwardly to my whole experience (both my mind's and
my body's), my mind can feel into my leg . . . It's simply a matter
of learning to listen to a different level of presence, realizing
that the silence within my paralysis isn't lost . . . When I truly
listen, I hear what exists before movement . . . what's present
before I enter the world through effort and action, before I
engage my will . . . I gain some form of energetic awareness — a
tingling, a feeling of movement, not outward but inward, a sense
of hum. It's a form of presence, and it subtly connects my mind
to my body.*[9]

This awareness was deeply restorative for Matthew, and he echoes my own experience when he says, "There are many possibilities for healing within the mind-body relationship. There is healing other than healing to walk again."[10] The healing journey never ends: you just have the chance to live it as fully as you can, moment by moment, day by day. It's never smooth, and, despite my twenty years of meditation, I often find my awareness wants to bounce away from my body when the pain is bad. But, like Matthew, I'm committed to the practice of returning to my body as fully as I can — despite the injuries and the pain — and finding rest, peace, and ease there. That's my life's work. As Matthew says, "I am still returning to my body and will do so for the rest of my life."[11]

HEALING TOWARD THE HUMAN CONDITION

The practice of mindfulness — resting more fully in the moment — has brought an unexpected gift. I've experienced a profound turnaround in which my life in its wholeness, including my pain, has become a point of connection with others. Fighting and running from my pain kept me preoccupied with myself, and that raised a wall of separation. There was no stillness and hence no inner space that could enable me to gaze over the parapet of myself and glimpse a radically different perspective on life. When that finally happened it was like turning 180 degrees — rather than moving *away* from life in search of a better existence, I turned back *toward* it. I'd felt like a lonely person in a wilderness, but the view is now full of color, variety, and other people.

I call this transformation "healing toward the human condition," and for me, it's the deepest healing of all. It has helped me take my place in humanity just as I am: flawed, yet alive, just like everyone else. It's such a relief to let go of the idea that I should be perfect and to see each moment as an opportunity for empathy and connectedness in which my pain and joy, my capacity to love and be loved, are reflected in others.

Wholeness is inclusive. If even the smallest part of you is excluded, then wholeness itself is fractured. If you exclude your pain and difficulties from your life by resisting them or expelling them into the cold of unawareness, you cannot be whole: you cannot heal or be happy in the deepest sense. But if you allow life in without resistance or clinging, you can be healthy and whole, no matter what kind of injury or disease process you may be living with. You can be like the wild geese in the following poem by Mary Oliver. No matter who you are, however lonely and desperate you may feel, "the world offers itself up to your imagination." Like the geese, you can "head home again" and announce "your place in the family of things."

Wild Geese

You do not have to be good.
You do not have to walk on your knees
for a hundred miles through the desert, repenting.
You only have to let the soft animal of your body
  love what it loves.
Tell me about despair, yours, and I will tell you mine.
Meanwhile the world goes on.
Meanwhile the sun and the clear pebbles of the rain
are moving across the landscapes,
over the prairies and the deep trees,
the mountains and the rivers.
Meanwhile the wild geese, high in the clean blue air,
are heading home again.
Whoever you are, no matter how lonely,
the world offers itself up to your imagination,
calls to you like the wild geese, harsh and exciting –
over and over announcing your place
in the family of things.[12]

MARY OLIVER

PART III

*

Coming Home to the Body

CHAPTER 7

The Breath

The morning wind spreads its fresh smell.
We must get up and take that in,
That wind that lets us live.
Breathe before it's gone.

RUMI[1]

BODY AWARENESS AS REHABILITATION

In a short story by James Joyce called "A Painful Case," a character named Mr. Duffy is described as "living at a little distance from his body."[2] That wonderful description evokes a way of living that's very familiar to me from the times when I'm not mindful. My ideas and willpower drive my actions; I'm aware of myself only from the neck up while the rest of my body feels very far away, as if covered by mist. Even if my body is crying out for attention, the cries seem to be in the distance, and I hope that if I ignore them they'll go away.

This section explores bringing mindfulness to the body, which is especially important for those of us living with pain and illness. Often the body is the last thing we want to be aware of, and so we develop habits that enable us to evade such awareness. This is an understandable response to living with a painful body, but it creates secondary suffering. A crucial role of mindfulness is to invite awareness back to the body as a kindly, gentle place of rest.

An evocative word for what happens when this connection is restored is *rehabilitation,* which means "to render fit again" or "to restore." It shares a root with the French verb *habiter,* meaning "to dwell," so rehabilitation could be seen as learning to live, or dwell, inside oneself again in order to restore well-being. [3] All the methods in this book are ways of reinhabiting the body with greater harmony and ease, no matter how painful the body may feel. Learning to live with the body rather than fighting *against* it is the path to rehabilitation and a richer, more satisfying quality of life.

One of the most effective ways to bring awareness into your body is to develop awareness of your breath. It's a constant presence and rhythm in your body, and every time you become aware of it, you naturally have a moment of body awareness. This is one of the reasons why we value it so highly at Breathworks.

WHAT IS THE BREATH?

The process we call breathing is one of the many things we take for granted. It flows in and out of the body in about eleven thousand cycles a day or four million cycles a year, and it is perhaps our most basic life-affirming activity. Breathing is a label for all the physical movements that cause air to flow in and out of the body. One way to think of the breath is as borrowed air.

The rhythm of respiration is echoed throughout nature — in the internal respiration of the cells, the ebb and flow of the tides, the waxing and waning of the moon, and the pulse of the seasons. Fish, birds, and even the most basic cellular life-forms follow the rhythm of respiration: taking in and giving back, moving up and down, in and out. Look at the pulsing movement of a jellyfish that glides through the sea by displacing water. Even plants have respiration that echoes our own. These natural rhythms also change endlessly: no two tides are exactly the same size or duration, and likewise our breath is continually varied within its basic rhythm, each breath having a unique quality.

Throughout history and in many cultures, breathing has been associated with health, consciousness, and spirit. For example, in the ancient Indian language of Sanskrit, *prana* is the life force coursing within us that is closely associated with the breath and only ceases at the moment of death. The breath is like a river running through a dry valley that gives life to everything it touches. By waking up to its beauty and mystery, you can learn to live in a painful body with dignity, vitality, and health.

The Anatomy of Breathing

The primary physical function of breathing is to supply oxygen to the body's cells, where it is used to chemically "burn" food, releasing energy that's fundamental to all of the body's functions. This creates carbon dioxide, a waste product that is released back into the atmosphere on the out-breath. Without oxygen, the cells die, which is why breathing is the first and last act of conscious life.

The complex biochemical process through which oxygen from the air feeds the cells starts when the in-breath is triggered by internal systems regulating the rate of respiration to maintain a stable level of oxygen and carbon dioxide in the blood. The big muscle of the central diaphragm flattens down, and the ribs expand, creating a partial vacuum in the chest cavity. As the air pressure in the chest is now lower than that in the atmosphere, air pours in, filling the lungs. It flows into tiny sacs in the lungs, where oxygen passes into the blood to be pumped around the body (see figure 3 on page 80). When it reaches the cells, it is released into the tissues and transformed into energy. Simultaneously, the waste product — carbon dioxide — is released from the cells into the blood, where it travels back through the circulatory system to the lungs. It is then released from the blood into the air sacs to pour out of the body on the out-breath when the diaphragm relaxes back into the chest, causing the lungs to deflate.

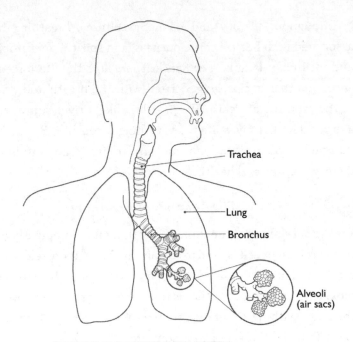

FIGURE 3: THE RESPIRATORY SYSTEM

The whole process is initiated by two groups of respiratory muscles: the primary muscles, which are essential for full breathing, and the accessory — or secondary — muscles. In optimal breathing the primary muscles do almost all the work. They're deeper and lower in the body and include the diaphragm, the intercostal muscles (which are between the ribs), and the deep abdominal muscles at the front of the belly. The accessory muscles — including the muscles in the neck, the shoulders, and the upper ribs — do about 20 percent of the work only.

The diaphragm is the most important primary respiratory muscle, and it is responsible for most respiratory effort. It is a large, dome-shaped muscle that rests inside the chest like a parachute or an umbrella. A central tendon at the top of the diaphragm sits just beneath the heart, with fibers radiating out like the panels of a parachute. They attach at the front to a little bone at the tip of the

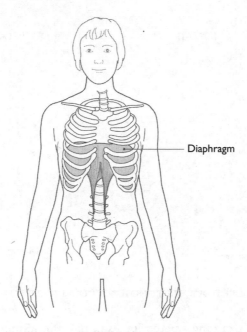

FIGURE 4: THE DIAPHRAGM

breastbone called the xiphoid process, and at the sides they attach to the insides of the lower ribs. At the back, two long tendons attach to the first four lumbar vertebrae of the spine to act like the handle of an umbrella (see figure 4). You may think that the breath only affects the front of the body, but these connections mean that the back of the body is also actively involved in breathing.

Whenever you breathe in, the diaphragm flattens and broadens; when you breathe out, it relaxes and billows back into the chest, resuming its natural dome shape (see figure 5 on page 82). It moves up and down in a regular, tireless rhythm. You can't feel this movement directly because the diaphragm lies so deep in the body, but you can infer it through its effects. Each time the diaphragm flattens on the in-breath it displaces the inner organs, causing the belly to swell outward and sideways. The organs are continually massaged, squeezed, and rolled by this movement, bathing them in new blood, fluids, and

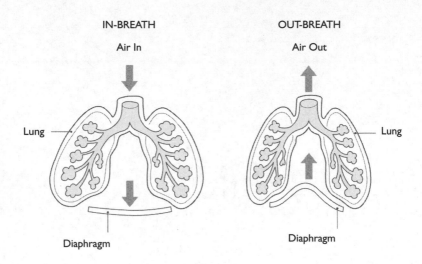

IN-BREATH   OUT-BREATH

Air In   Air Out

Lung   Lung

Diaphragm   Diaphragm

FIGURE 5: DIAPHRAGM MOVEMENT DURING BREATH CYCLE

oxygen and draining waste. For example, the kidneys slide up and down beside the spine up to one-and-a-half inches with each breath cycle.[4] The whole spine is simultaneously rocked and cradled.

This is a description of full-bodied breathing, sometimes called diaphragmatic breathing, which stimulates the whole body and deeply affects our sense of well-being. If you have pain, your breathing will probably be inhibited in some way, but over time, simply bringing awareness to the inhibition with an understanding of basic anatomy can gently release any patterns of holding. This allows your awareness to drop deep within the body and restores optimal, health-giving breathing patterns.

Why Is Breath Awareness So Important?

My colleagues and I chose the name "Breathworks" for our mindfulness-based pain-management program because we believe that awareness of the breath *works* as a powerful aid to cultivating mindfulness, coming home to the body, and easing secondary suffering. It runs as a thread through our approach, unifying the various practices. Breath awareness helps in several ways:

- The breath is a *helpful and simple focus of awareness* in cultivating mindfulness.
- It *anchors awareness in the body.* You only directly know the breath through the body's sensations and movements. When you feel the quality and texture of each breath, your awareness naturally becomes grounded in the body.
- It *anchors awareness in the present moment.* Breath awareness is always present-moment awareness because you can only perceive the breath as it affects the body right now. A past or a future breath is just an idea.
- It's a *tool for managing reactions to pain, illness, and stress.* When you avoid or resist pain or discomfort, the tendency is to hold the breath or inhibit its flow. Everyone does this under stress, but in the case of a chronic condition, inhibiting the breath becomes a habit that unwittingly creates more pain and tension. A vicious cycle can start in which chronic pain leads to tension, which brings more pain, resulting in more tension. Breathing *in* to the experience of pain interrupts this cycle, and gradually the tension reduces.

❋ **LESLEY**

Four times a year Lesley is part of a team providing weekend breaks for people who care for disabled parents or children. It's hard work cooking, cleaning, doing dishes, and so on. When her back pain gets really bad she uses her breath to ease the tension that's built up around the pain. She can actually feel the tension releasing, so she is left with just the initial pain without any extras. She sees the pain as changing from moment to moment, and knowing that at times the pain will ease up is enough to get her through the day.

Imaginatively directing your breathing *toward* the pain naturally undermines the habit of inhibiting the breath, and it can be a great relief to let go and relax on the out-breath. The primary pain may not change, but as you relax the secondary layers of tension and resistance begin to dissolve. This is also true of emotional distress — feeling upset is often associated with contracted breath. Calm and peacefulness naturally arise when you become aware of this tendency and breathe *in* to emotional tension and let go on the out-breath.

THE SPIRIT OF INQUIRY

A way to start becoming familiar with the breath as a felt experience in the body is through short "breath inquiries" that direct your awareness to the sensations of breathing in an uncomplicated way, with curiosity, leaving aside ideas of whether you're doing it right.[5] (Audio versions of the three inquiries in this chapter are available from soundstrue.com/burch.)

> **BREATH INQUIRY 1: TENSION AND THE BREATH**
> Clench your fist and notice what happens to the breath. You'll probably find that you hold the breath and that it feels frozen in the abdomen. Now relax around your breath and breathe into the sensations of clenching. Can you notice how your fist relaxes a little as well?

The tendency of the breath to freeze in response to the fist mirrors the way we tend to inhibit the breath in response to pain. The inquiry also shows how you can use the breath to break the pain/tension cycle by undoing the habit of holding the breath against pain, which causes extra tension.

The habit of inhibiting the breath can manifest as shallow breathing, frozen breathing, overbreathing, rushing the breath, and so on.[6] Through mindfulness and breath awareness you can notice any habits such as these and then let go and soften around the breath. You may also notice that you quickly revert to inhibiting and tightening the breath — that's the way habits work. Never mind: the practice is to soften this tension with a gentle attitude each time you notice it. Gradually you can learn new habits of breathing more deeply and with greater relaxation.

BREATH INQUIRY 2: THE BASIC BREATH

Adopt a comfortable posture lying down or sitting in a chair. Now close your eyes and tune in to the breath without judging or altering it, and place your hand on the part of your body that moves most when you breathe. If you notice your chest moving more than your abdomen, it means your breathing is a little shallow.

Now place your hands on your abdomen just below the rib cage with the middle fingers of each hand lightly touching. Let your abdomen move freely as the diaphragm flattens down inside the body and then relaxes back with each breath cycle. Allow this to happen without effort, just letting the natural breath breathe without inhibition, finding its own rhythm. Let go of ideas of right or wrong and tune in to what's happening with receptivity and curiosity. See if you can sense the abdominal muscles softening and releasing under your hands.

Notice what else is happening in your body: how the tips of your fingers move slightly apart as you breathe in, and come together again as you breathe out. Note any tension in your chest, throat, or abdomen; this is normal for most of us and will subside as you begin to breathe more optimally. You might also notice some unusual sensations or little muscle twitches as you release tension. These should settle down over time.

Many people find this inquiry easiest to do lying down. You can also experiment with other postures and notice the quality of your breath when you're sitting, standing, or lying.

Back Breathing

Most of us associate the breath with the chest and front of the body — perhaps because our eyes look forward we are more attuned to the front than the back of the body. But the ribs and the lungs form part of the back of the body as well as the front, and the spine also moves with the breath. Paying attention to the movement of the "back breath" stimulates the parasympathetic part of the autonomic nervous system associated with calm, rest, and relaxation.[7] It broadens and deepens your sense of the body, allows awareness to drop more deeply into it, and counters the tendency to race on to the next thing.

QUALITIES OF OPTIMAL, FULL-BODY BREATHING

Stop moving to become still
And the stillness will move.
— ZEN POEM[8]

Oscillation

When the natural breath flows through the body there may be a lovely sense of quietness, but never total stillness. Full-body breathing undulates and oscillates through the body, like waves rising and falling on the ocean. On the in-breath this movement ripples from the center of the body to the pores of the skin, and then dissolves back to the center on the out-breath. The movement is like that of a flower that blooms and then enfolds itself.[9]

Diaphragm

The whole breathing process is led by the movement of the central diaphragm. Unlike the secondary muscles that are higher in the body and become tense and strained if they take over leading the breathing process, the diaphragm never tires. That's why diaphragmatic breathing is easy and relaxing.

Effortlessness

When you're at rest and breathing optimally, each breath arises naturally and without any willed effort. The movement of the diaphragm naturally initiates the in-breath, but the out-breath takes place without any muscular effort at all. This is simply the result of the diaphragm relaxing and resuming its dome shape, causing air to pour out of the lungs like a deflating balloon. It's important not to force the out-breath, nor to rush the in-breath. *Let the breath breathe itself.* Full-body breathing is always relaxing.

Two/Three/Pause Rhythm

Optimal full-body breathing is naturally calm and regular without being mechanical. It's normal for the inhalation to last about two seconds and the exhalation to last about three seconds, followed by a pause. Within this rhythm the breath is endlessly varied, continually adapting to the changing emotional, mental, and physical conditions of each moment.

Drink from the Well of the Pause

It's fascinating to explore the pause between the end of the out-breath and the beginning of the in-breath. The body moves continually with the breath, but there's a point of balance when the out-breath naturally exhausts its momentum and fades into stillness. Then comes a moment of hovering anticipation, a vibration that gathers into the next in-breath.

When a receding wave flows down a beach toward the sea, the water pauses before gathering into a fresh wave that flows back up the beach. A wave drinks from the ocean just as a new breath drinks from the air. If you disrupt the rhythm by rushing on to the next breath, you will inhibit the precious moment of "drinking air" from which the new breath is born, thus disturbing the breathing process.

▶ BREATH INQUIRY 3: WHOLE-BODY BREATHING

You can do this inquiry sitting or lying down, whichever is most comfortable and relaxing.

INTRODUCTION

Loosen any tight clothing and allow your body to be supported by the earth. Let the weight of the body sink downward, so that your awareness settles deep in the body. Engage in this inquiry with a spirit of kindly curiosity.

ABDOMEN

Take your awareness to the abdominal area—the whole soft front of the body from the pelvis up to the base of the ribs and the tip of the sternum. Tune in to the movements of the abdomen as you breathe. Allow it to swell to the front and the sides, broadening and opening on the in-breath, gently subsiding on the out-breath. Sense how the internal organs are rolled and massaged by these movements.

TENSING AND RELEASING

Sometimes it can be hard to tell if your breathing is relaxed, so experiment with drawing in the abdomen and holding it for a few breaths, then let go completely on the out-breath. You may find that you now want to take a deeper in-breath; if so, let the air flow freely into the body and follow it with your awareness. Play around with this tensing, releasing, and deeper breathing a few times in your own way until you can tell the difference between holding and releasing, then allow the breath to return to its own rhythm, letting the belly be soft. Let all the movements happen of their own accord as the breath breathes itself. Allow each exhalation to come to an end effortlessly and allow the next in-breath to naturally arise.

PELVIC FLOOR

Now take your awareness to the pelvic floor—the diamond-shaped area between the pubic bone and the tailbone. Notice any movement that echoes the movement of the diaphragm and other muscles.

To detect any holding, tighten the anus and the buttocks. Now draw in the pelvic floor, holding it in for a few breaths, then completely let go, allowing the next in-breath to be full and deep. Repeat this a few times in your own way, then let the movement settle. Notice how the pelvic floor broadens and opens on the in-breath and tones and retracts—more gently than a muscular contraction—on the out-breath. You can also sense this release in the pelvic floor if you let your jaw hang open and sigh slightly as you breathe, or imagine that a light bulb in the pelvic floor glows on the in-breath and dims on the out-breath.

SACRUM AND LOWER BACK
Now take your awareness to the back of the body and feel the sacrum—the triangular bone at the base of the spine. The sacrum takes most of your weight when you're lying down, so you'll feel pressure on it. Notice any movement in this area, perhaps a sense of the weight slightly changing as you breathe. Broaden your awareness to include the lower back and sense the slight rocking of the pelvis with the breath. Notice how the lower back arches away from the floor on the inhalation and flattens and lengthens against it on the exhalation. These are subtle movements, like an ocean swell. If you can't feel anything, see if you can imagine this gentle rocking.

The pelvic floor, sacrum, and lower back are the roots of the natural breath. Allowing the breath to drop deep in the body so they move freely brings calm and release and reduces tension higher in the body.

SPINE
Starting with awareness of the sacrum and the tailbone at the bottom of the spine, gradually take your awareness up the spine, vertebra by vertebra, through the lower, middle, and upper spine to the point where the neck meets the skull. All along the spine, interlocking bones affect one another in delicate and complex ways. Imagine they are like bits of driftwood floating on the sea, strung together by the spinal cord. They float up on the in-breath and float down on the out-breath,

without resistance or inhibition, rocked and cradled by the swell of the breath. Notice the broadness of the back. With each in-breath it broadens and opens, sinking back down as you breathe out.

SHOULDERS

Now take your awareness to your shoulders and arms. Allow the arms to rest on the floor with the hands palm upward, if that's comfortable; this allows the shoulders to respond to the breath. Look for the gentle movement of the shoulders on the inhalation that starts at the breastbone and flows across each collarbone to the shoulder sockets. Notice how the arms rotate slightly outward in the shoulder sockets on the in-breath and then release back. Rest for a few moments, sense the flow of movement through the shoulders and arms, and inhabit those movements with your awareness without changing or altering the breath. Let the breath breathe itself, and rest within its gentle movement.

THROAT

Now feel the throat and imagine it is soft and open, offering no inhibition to the flow of air. Anxiety or tension can bring strain to this area, especially if it's associated with communication. If you notice tension, see if you can let the breath flow freely through the throat and release any holding.

FULL-BODY BREATHING

Broadening out your awareness, allow a sense of softness to spread through the body with the breath: soft vocal cords and throat, soft belly, soft buttocks, soft pelvic floor, soft back and shoulders, soft face and hands. Let the body be free and open as it's rocked and cradled by the breath—still, yet continually moving. See if you can sense tiny rocking movements in the hands and feet as the breath ripples out to the edges of the body.

Imagine the skin is like a knitted sheath covering the body, perhaps noticing the sensations of your clothes against your skin. On the in-breath, feel the strands of this sheath expand and create space; on the out-breath, feel them condense.

CONCLUSION

Gradually draw this inquiry to a close. Become aware of sounds, as well as the weight and mass of your body. As you consider beginning to move, form an intention to maintain this full-body breathing and see if you can move *with* the breath rather than guarding against it. If you're lying down, be careful not to strain your back and neck as you move—roll on to one side, if this is comfortable, before coming upright. Make sure your head follows your spine upright, naturally uncurling.

Breath awareness is a simple technique, but many people find that learning to work with the breath, using it to soften resistance and holding, has a profound effect on their quality of life and overall experience of suffering.

EMMA

Recently, when my client Emma went to a concert, she managed to sit for the whole program, enjoying every moment. As she sat down with her friends, she closed her eyes and brought her awareness to her breath. She was experiencing a flare-up of the pain caused by her chronic illness, and she noticed the tension in her body, but she breathed in toward this and felt her neck and shoulders relax.

As she listened to the music, she stayed aware of the movement of the breath in her body. She imagined she was inhaling the music on the in-breath and exhaling it on the out-breath. The pain and discomfort were still there, but simply by attending to the music and her breath, it became just a part of her experience. When the pain grew intense, she breathed the music into the pain and continued to let go on the out-breath. After two hours, the last notes of Dvorak's "New World" Symphony drifted away, and she became aware of the sounds of the audience and opened her eyes. Despite her pain, she'd been entranced.

CHAPTER 8

Mindful Movement

Your grief for what you've lost lifts a mirror
up to where you're bravely working.
Expecting the worst, you look, and instead,
here's the joyful face you've been wanting to see.
Your hand opens and closes and opens and closes.
If it were always a fist or always stretched open,
you would be paralyzed.
Your deepest presence is in every small contracting
and expanding,
the two as beautifully balanced and coordinated
as bird wings.

RUMI[1]

I f you want to use mindfulness to help you live well with pain, illness, or stress, then it's important to develop the body's flexibility and strength by moving it within the limits of your physical capacity. This reverses any habits of restricting your movement that may have developed in your efforts to avoid pain, from inhibiting your breath to avoiding any strenuous movement at all. Muscles that don't move become muscles that *can't* move, and a vicious cycle may start as stiffness and weakness lead to tension and pain, prompting even more stiffness. A mindful approach to movement can turn this around. As you develop strength and flexibility, you'll gradually regain confidence in your ability to move.

✳ ALISON

Alison damaged her leg in a devastating car accident and was in the hospital and then housebound for a long time. She'd been still for such a long time that she was rigid and frightened, and any movement was painful. When she first tried mindful movement, it was good just to stretch her body and think, *It's okay, I'll just do what I can manage without pushing.*

At Breathworks we've developed a comprehensive sequence of movements based on yoga and Pilates that are suitable for people living with pain and illness (see page 271). Here, I'll introduce the basic principles and a range of movements for you to start with. I've personally found a daily movement program to be invaluable for my health and well-being; I go swimming twice a week and regularly do a sequence of the mindful movements. This helps me maintain a level of fitness, but it quickly dwindles if I don't practice mindful movement for a few days.

MOVING WITH THE BREATH

In the previous chapter we saw that even when you lie down quietly, breathing causes a ceaseless, rhythmic movement. Motion is natural to the body and its systems — the musculoskeletal, digestive, circulatory, immune, nervous, and endocrine — thrive on it. Even the bone cells are in a constant state of movement as they replenish themselves, and the entire skeleton is completely replaced every seven to ten years.

✳ CHARLOTTE

Charlotte experiences a lot of pain due to a hypermobility syndrome, but she's devoted to the mindful movements.

When I'm too still I feel like a concrete block. I like being active and getting to know my body in a subtle way, listening to it and letting it guide me, so the mindful movements are great for me. My joints love movement; it's what they need. Paying careful attention as I move helps me bring awareness to normal movements like opening a door or lifting a kettle, and that changes my whole experience.

The key to the movements in this chapter is the principle that movement itself is natural and grows from the breath. You could even see this kind of movement as "breath in action." You'll need to let the body find its natural flow, rhythm, and balance and then extend that into specific postures. When movement grows from the natural breath, the body's energy flows more freely, and tension releases, bringing fluidity to your whole physical, mental, and emotional experience. If you notice your breath is inhibited, just pause, explore what that feels like, and reconnect with the breath.

These movements are primarily aimed at helping you to become mindful by developing the *quality* of your attention as you move. Becoming sensitive to your body's sensations allows you to inhabit it more deeply and feel more relaxed, grounded, and alive. If you practice regularly you'll also grow stronger and more flexible. However, we don't call the mindful movements "exercises" because many people associate physical exercises solely with achieving results such as improved mobility. The focus here is on bringing awareness to the *process* of movement. This will help you learn useful new habits that you can take into daily activities.

Posture

Some of the movements introduced here are carried out from a lying position, while others are done sitting or standing. This offers different options for people with varying physical capacities. If you can get down on the floor, I recommend you begin with the movements that are done lying down. Your mindfulness will naturally deepen if you can give the weight of your body to the earth, free from the compression of gravity. You'll probably find it easier to release around the spine and relax around the breath, especially if your condition means that an upright position aggravates structural misalignments and muscle imbalances.

What If There Are Some Movements That You Can't Do?

If you are unable to manage all the movements, don't worry. Do whichever ones you can. You can also adapt them according to your particular
health condition or disability. The main thing is to gradually extend the
range of your movement and become sensitive to your body's movement
as an expression of the rhythm of the breath. You can always do this,
even if your fitness and flexibility are limited. In the case of movements
you can't manage, it may help to visualize them. Research shows this can
improve your fitness and health, and it can also be very enjoyable.[2]

Safety

These movements are safe for everyone if they're practiced with care
and you leave out any that are unsuitable for your injury or disability.
If you are at all uncertain, consult your health professional. The key is
mindfulness: being curious and sensitive to how your body feels with
each movement rather than pushing it. It's easy to think that you
should move in a certain way — and then injure yourself — instead of
putting your effort into inhabiting the body deeply and with kindly
curiosity. You can take satisfaction in developing awareness in even
the smallest movements.

If you're fit, the movements may seem too simple for you. But even
the simplest activities are opportunities to deepen your awareness.
Sometimes the quieter movements help cultivate an exquisite and
delicate sensitivity of awareness.

Soft and Hard Edges

If you are inclined to push yourself, you'll need to watch out for that tendency as you practice these movements. Then again, if you're scared of moving in daily life, you'll probably benefit from asking more of yourself. A useful way to gauge if you're stretching your capacities without overdoing it is to work within your *hard* and *soft* edges.

The *soft edge* is the point at which you first feel sensations of stretch or challenge; for example, when you bend the knee, the soft edge is the point at which you first feel a sensation of stretch and compression. Finding this soft edge requires sensitivity. Without working slowly and mindfully it's easy to quickly move past it without noticing.

The *hard edge* is the last point of movement before strain occurs. Going beyond this point risks injury. You'll know if you move beyond the hard edge because you'll feel you're forcing that part of your body, and it may even tremble.

Working Between the Hard and Soft Edges Is Ideal

Your body will benefit most from these movements when you work between the soft and hard edges so that the area involved in the movement is mobilized but not strained. See if your tendency is toward doing too much or not enough, and then find the point of balance. The most creative place to work is usually a moderate stretch that can be sustained, not an intense one that you can't hold for long. Your edges will change from day to day and also as you grow stronger and more flexible.

Different Sorts of Pains to Watch Out For

Sometimes it can be hard to know which aches and pains mean you need to be careful and which are a healthy sign of stretching. Feeling a dull ache, tiredness in the muscles, or stretch in the tissues is natural and lessens over time, but if you notice electrical, nervy, or sharp sensations, reduce the range of the movement or stop altogether. It's good to err toward caution, and if you aren't sure, seek advice from a health practitioner.

Points to Remember

- Repeat each movement a few times with an attitude of play and curiosity. See if you can drop into a deep awareness of the breath as you move, allowing the breath to lead the pace of the movement rather than forcing it or rushing through the movements.
- Always do symmetrical movements on both sides of the body, but bear in mind this may feel different on either side. If you pause between sides, often the one you've moved feels more alive and awake.
- If you're working with an injury, it's usually helpful to do the less challenged side first.
- Practicing the movements regularly can bring surprising progress even if you seem to be doing very little in any one session.
- Always leave a few minutes at the end of a session to relax completely in a comfortable position and to give your body and mind time to assimilate the effects.

❋ **ANNIE**

I injured my neck a couple of years ago, and I've found it hard to accept, but mindful movement shows me that I still have a body and I want to be aware of it. It's a great way to be kind to myself instead of getting angry and frustrated. In other exercises, the emphasis is on trying to get somewhere. That's important, too, but I become unwilling to experience my body in the present. The mindful movements calm me down; they've also helped me enjoy swimming more. I find it very meditative now and enjoy the feeling of the different strokes rather than just counting the number of lengths I've done.

Other Forms of Exercise

As you engage with these movements you may find your interest is stimulated to explore other forms of exercise and movement. If so, I suggest you look for a skilled movement instructor and obtain individual guidance—it could be in yoga, Pilates, tai chi, or qigong—or you might join a gym or go swimming. What's important is that you keep the body moving, build health and vitality while using the opportunity to develop mindfulness, and enjoy it!

Free Movement

Another way to explore moving the body is through free movement. Choose a favorite piece of music, preferably one that's calm, and find a position—lying, sitting, or standing—in which you'll be comfortable and able to move. Make sure you have a clear space to move in and start by really feeling the music and breathing with it. Gently allow the body to follow the music in movement with no set form. I love doing this, and it seems to open my body very deeply. I like to do it lying on the floor, stretching and releasing different joints and muscles in a gentle and sensuous way.

Recently I introduced this technique in a course for people with pain. At one point I looked around the room and the participants were moving in all sorts of fluid ways, mostly maintaining close contact with the floor for support, utterly absorbed in the music and activity. One was eighty-four, another was recovering from cancer treatment, while a third was recovering from long-term chronic fatigue. They were all delighted to find such a pleasurable way to move, free from self-consciousness and inhibition.

THE MINDFUL MOVEMENTS

All that's important is this one moment in movement. Make the moment important, vital, and worth living. Don't let it slip away unnoticed and unused.

MARTHA GRAHAM (CHOREOGRAPHER)

MOVEMENTS FROM LYING DOWN

Supporting the Head and Neck

It's important to maintain the neck and head in a neutral position when lying on your back. Use a firm cushion or folded blanket for support. Experiment to find a height that's neither too low, overstretching the front of the neck (see figure 6a), nor too high, overstretching the back of the neck (see figure 6b). The optimum position (see figure 6c) is when the forehead is slightly higher than the chin, allowing freedom in the neck by maintaining its natural curve.

This neck support is also recommended if lying down to do Breath Inquiry 3 in chapter 7 (see page 88) and the body scan and meditation practices introduced in part 5.

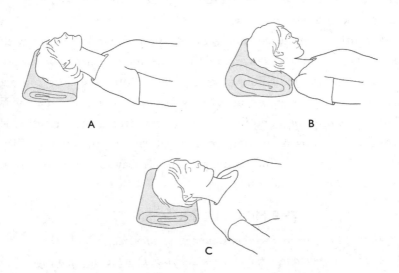

FIGURE 6: SUPPORT FOR THE NECK AND HEAD

Beginning: The Breathing Body

Lie on your back, supporting your head as shown, and take a few minutes to engage with the movements of the natural breath. To ease any strain on your back, raise your knees so your feet are flat on the floor (see figure 7a). Alternatively, place a bolster, rolled blanket, or cushions under your lower thighs and knees (see figure 7b). Otherwise, lie with your legs outstretched (see figure 7c).

Place your hands on your body and notice the movement as your breath rises and falls. Notice the texture, depth, length, and ease of your breath; let go of what you think *should* be happening and tune in to your actual experience of the breath. For a few breaths gently exhale through your mouth, making a soft "ah" sound. Inhale normally through your nose. This helps to relax the body and deepens the breath. Extend your awareness to include sensations, feelings, and thoughts as they arise and pass away.

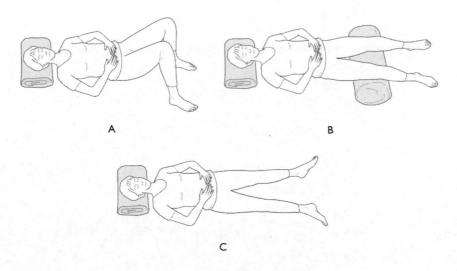

A

B

C

FIGURE 7: THE BREATHING BODY

Moving with the Breath

In some of the following movements I suggest a specific way of moving with the breath; in others you can experiment to see which phase of the breathing best supports the movement.

Opening Hands

Rest one hand on the floor, palm upward, while the other rests on your body (see figure 8a). Guided by the breath, open and close the outstretched hand so that the movement mirrors the expanding and subsiding of the breath (see figure 8b). See if your hand's movements can be led by the breath's natural rhythm. Repeat with the other hand and then both hands at the same time.

Core Stability

In all the movements that follow, see if you can engage the muscles that create your core stability in your abdomen and lower back before initiating the movement, especially when moving the legs or abdomen.

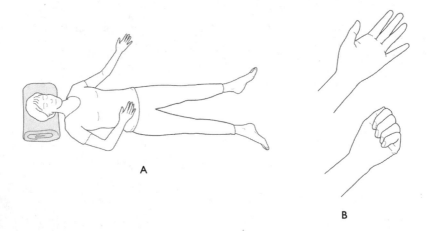

A

B

FIGURE 8: MOVING HANDS WITH THE BREATH

This avoids straining the lower back. Before each movement, imagine the base of your spine is lengthening away from the upper spine so that the lower back draws down toward the floor with the spine long and the pelvis stable. This gently draws your abdomen back toward the spine and engages the abdominal muscles.

Leg Cradle

Lying on your back, gently bend your knees so your feet rest on the floor (refer back to figure 7a). Keeping one foot on the floor, engage the core stability muscles by lengthening through the spine, and gently ease the other leg toward your chest. Hold it in a way that's comfortable, probably behind the back of the thigh or at the top of the shin (see figure 9a). If this creates too much strain, support the leg by holding a belt or strap behind the thigh (see figure 9b). Gently move the leg in and out, and circle it from the hip to stretch and move the hip and lower back. Try to keep the pelvis stable as you move the leg. Remember to let the rhythm of the movements follow the natural breath, and experiment within your range of movement. See if you can let the breath be free rather than contracting against it.

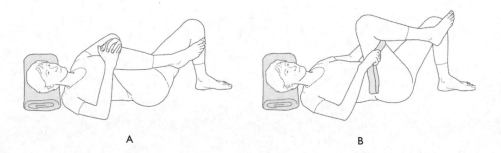

A   B

FIGURE 9: LEG CRADLE

Leg Cradle — Both Legs

Engaging the core stability muscles by lengthening through the spine, ease both thighs toward your chest — slowly, one leg at a time — and lightly hold your legs (use a strap, if necessary). Gently rock from side to side to massage the lower back (your knees can be together or apart, whichever is most comfortable).

Variation 1: Breath Echo

Being guided by the in-breath, allow your legs to gently ease away from your chest as you slightly straighten the arms. Exhaling, bend your arms and ease your thighs back toward your chest. After a while, stop making an effort to move and feel the echo of the movement as your body oscillates in time with the natural breath (see figure 10).

Variation 2: Swimming

Holding each leg separately in a way that's comfortable, circle your legs from the hips in opposite directions to make a swimming movement, as if you're doing the breaststroke. After a while, reverse the direction (see figure 11). This brings movement into the hips and decompresses the lower spine, releasing tension and keeping it mobile. If you have a

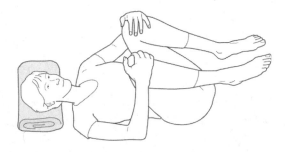

FIGURE 10: BREATH ECHO

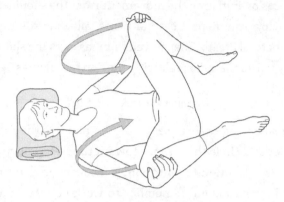

FIGURE 11: SWIMMING

painful lower back, try keeping the tips of your big toes lightly touching as you circle the legs — this provides more stability in the pelvis. You can also do the movement without involving the arms, if you find this easier.

Side-Lying Chair Movements

The next two movements are a sequence in which you lie on your side, so do them on one side and then the other. Place your thighs at 90 degrees to your spine and your lower legs at 90 degrees to your thighs, as if sitting on a chair. A bolster or cushion placed between your legs can give added comfort and stabilize the pelvis and lower back. Add folded blankets wide enough to support your head as you roll sideways a little. Make sure they're the right height and the neck is supported, not strained.

Variation 1: Shoulder Rock

From the side-lying chair pose, extend your arms and bring your palms together. Keeping both arms straight, slide your top arm forward and backward over the lower one, no more than a hand length. Focus on initiating the movement from the shoulder blade area of the moving arm. Repeat several times, allowing the rhythm to be led by the natural breath. This movement massages the shoulder blades and gently twists the spine, releasing tension (see figures 12a and 12b).

Variation 2: Clock Arm Circle

From the side-lying chair pose, bring the hand of the top arm onto its shoulder and circle the arm up toward the head, moving from the shoulder. Pay attention to your body's feedback in determining how far to circle the arm, and remember to work between your soft and hard edges. When you reach the hard edge, bring the arm back to the starting position. Some people are able to circle the arm fully; others find this too much, so explore what's best for you. Allow the head and

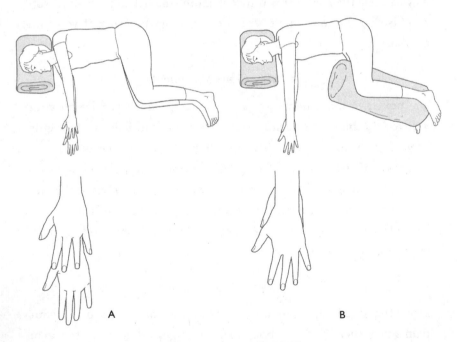

A   B

FIGURE 12: SHOULDER ROCK

torso to follow the arm, being led by the rhythm of the breath, and take the spine into a gentle twist (see figure 13). Keep your nose and chin in line with your sternum, or breastbone, as your arm rotates, to avoid overtwisting the neck. Many people find it helps to let the top leg lift away from the lower leg as the arm circles. Place a cushion between the legs if this feels more comfortable. Between sides, take a few moments to lie on your back and feel the different sensations in the two sides of the body.

This movement releases tension and brings mobility and freedom into the shoulders. As a gentle spinal twist it also helps to release the muscles around the spine and to stimulate the abdominal organs.

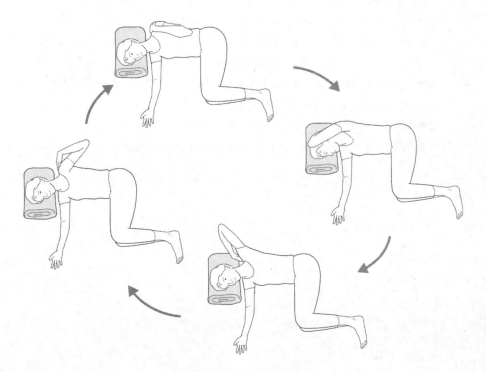

FIGURE 13: CLOCK ARM CIRCLE

Gentle Spinal Twist

Lie on your back with your head supported, arms out in line with your shoulders, palms up, and feet wide apart (see figure 14a). Coordinate your movements with the breath, moving on the exhalation and pausing on the inhalation. Remember to engage your core stability muscles each time you move by gently drawing in the abdomen and lengthening through the spine to provide support for the lower back.

Exhaling, take both legs gently to one side. Pause there as an inhalation naturally arises, and on the next out-breath bring the legs back to center. Pause again and inhale. On the next exhalation, take both legs to the other side and pause there, inhaling before returning to center with the next out-breath. Continue, allowing the movement to be led by the breath. If the twist feels too strong, put cushions by the legs to rest on when you take them to the side. After a while let the head and neck join in with the twist. When you take the legs to each side, gently turn the head away from the legs (see figure 14b). As the legs come back to center, bring the head to center as well. After a few repetitions, hold each side for a few breaths — or longer if this feels good. This movement releases and relaxes the whole body.

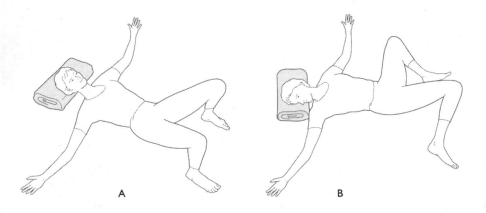

A   B

FIGURE 14: GENTLE SPINAL TWIST

Relaxation to End

Ease your thighs toward your chest (see figure 15a) before extending the legs and *relaxing*. Have a bolster or cushions under the legs if that's more comfortable (see figure 15b). Feel the sensations in your body and notice the quality and movement of your breath, as well as the flow of your feelings and thoughts.

MOVEMENTS FROM SITTING

These movements can be done sitting on a straight-backed chair and some may also be carried out from standing with the feet hip-width apart, keeping the knees soft. The principles of moving with the breath still apply. Relax your body into gravity and allow it to be supported by the earth. If you're sitting, refer to chapter 12 for guidance on maintaining a stable pelvis and an upright spine in a sitting posture (see also pages 157–159).

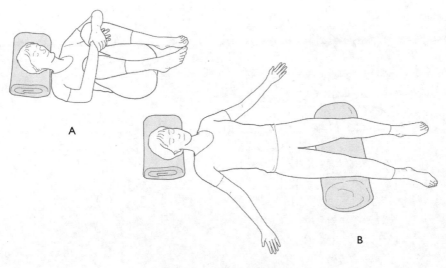

A

B

FIGURE 15: RELAXATION

Sequence 1 — Hands and Arms

Opening Hands

This is a sitting version of Opening Hands. If you're sitting, rest the backs of your hands lightly on your thighs (see figure 16a); if standing, let your arms hang loosely by your sides. Guided by the breath, open and close one hand so that the movement mirrors the expanding and subsiding of the breath (see figure 16b). Let the movement of your hand be led by the breath's natural rhythm. Repeat with the other hand and then move both hands together.

Prayer Hands

Sitting or standing, bring your hands in front of your chest with the palms and fingers pressed lightly together (see figure 17a). Move your

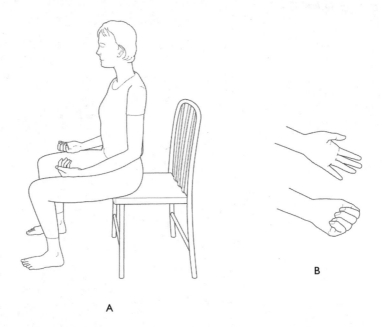

B

A

FIGURE 16: OPENING HANDS

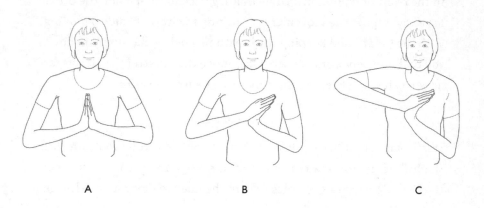

A   B   C

FIGURE 17: PRAYER HANDS

hands from side to side, feeling the movement in the wrists (see figure 17b). After a few cycles, keeping the heels of the hands together, raise the elbow of the upper arm as you move the hands to each side, keeping the shoulders relaxed (see figure 17c). Let the hands move to the sides on the out-breath and return to the center with each in-breath.

Now allow both arms to hang loosely by the sides of your body, making sure you keep the spine upright and the pelvis in a neutral position. Shake the arms lightly and relax the fingers, hands, wrists, elbows, and shoulders in a loose movement.

Sequence 2 — Feet and Legs

These movements are done from a sitting position.

Sliding Foot 1

With feet flat on the floor, rest your hands lightly on the thighs. Slowly slide one foot away from the chair, keeping the heel, ball of your foot, and toes in contact with the floor (see figure 18). You'll feel a stretch in the front of your ankle. Draw that leg back in, then slide the other leg away; repeat the movement. Continue to alternate sides, moving with the breath and keeping the breath relaxed. Make sure you don't roll back the pelvis and slouch. Only move the outstretched leg as far as you can while keeping the pelvis in a neutral position.

Sliding Foot 2

This is similar to Sliding Foot 1, but as you slide your foot out, lift the ball of the foot away from the floor, so you rest your weight on the heel. Gently draw the toes toward the knee to flex your ankle (see figure 19).

Foot Sway

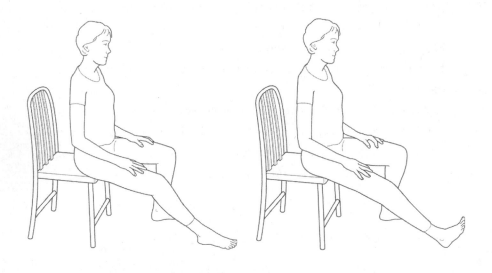

FIGURE 18: SLIDING FOOT 1   FIGURE 19: SLIDING FOOT 2

Now rest the weight of your extended leg on the heel of your foot with the knee soft and slightly bent. Gently sway the toes from side to side, feeling movement in the ankle. Allow the whole leg to relax and rock a little from side to side, releasing from the hip and following the movement of your foot. You may find it helpful to lightly hold the side of the chair for support (see figures 20a–c). Experiment with moving with the breath.

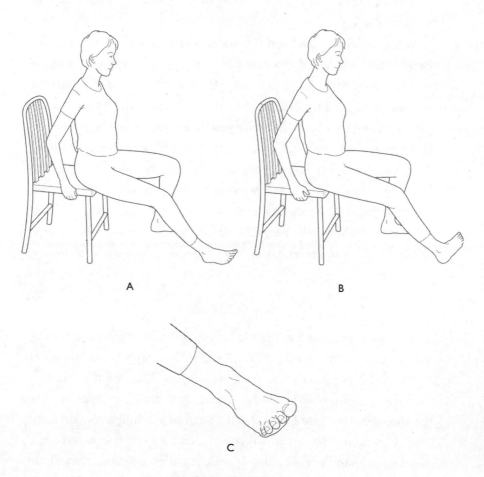

A   B

C

FIGURE 20: FOOT SWAY

Sequence 3 — Torso, Shoulders, and Upper Body

Gentle Twist

The movement is done in a sitting position. Sit forward on the chair, so the spine is upright, following its natural curves. To help you get a sense of lift through the spine, place your hands on your thighs and gently push down, lifting the heart away from the navel (see figures 21a and 21b). Be careful not to force and strain, making sure you keep your arms and shoulders soft.

With the legs parallel and hip-width apart, face forward with one hand placed on top of the other in your lap, keeping your fingers soft (see figures 21c and 21d). Leave the bottom hand in the starting position and slide the top hand to one side until the fingertips are just touching (see figure 21e). As you do so, turn the whole torso in the direction of the hand movement. You will probably turn about 45 degrees and feel a gentle spinal twist (see figure 21f). Slide the hands back into the starting position and repeat the movement on the other side. Do this movement a few times on each side, allowing the pace to be led by the natural breath. As you turn your torso, keep the nose, chin, and sternum in line so you don't overtwist the spine and neck.

Shoulder Rolls

If you're sitting, rest your hands lightly on your thighs; if standing, let the arms hang loosely by your sides. Gently draw one shoulder up toward the ear on the same side (see figure 22a), roll the shoulder round and down toward the back, and then draw it forward to the starting position (see figure 22b). Continue circling a few times in this way, then reverse the direction. Don't strain; the movements can be small and precise. Repeat on the other side, and then circle both shoulders together (see figures 22c–e). Be careful not to inhibit

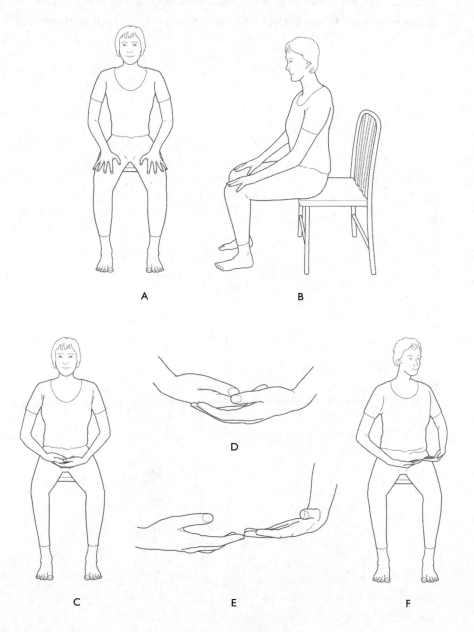

FIGURE 21: GENTLE TWIST

or hold your breath as you do this movement: see if you can move *with* the breath. Pause at the end to feel the effect of the movement.

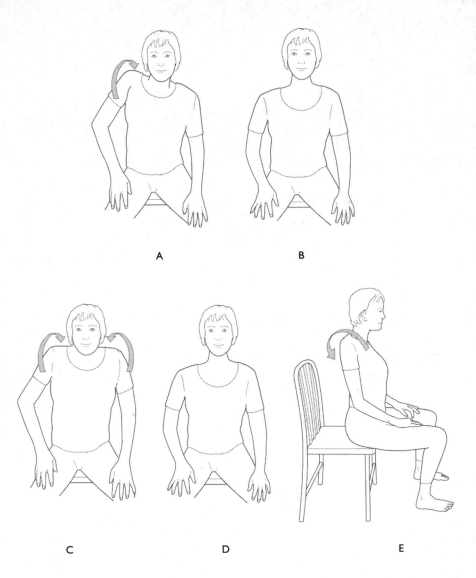

FIGURE 22: SHOULDER ROLLS

Shoulder Circles

This is a sitting version of Clock Arm Circle. Place one hand on your shoulder and bring the elbow forward and upward; continue to move the elbow around the shoulder in a full circle (see figures 23 a–d). If your shoulder is stiff or injured, make it a smaller movement in a

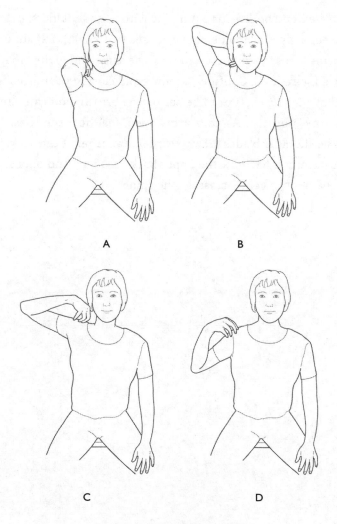

A   B

C   D

FIGURE 23: SHOULDER CIRCLES

semicircle, or just work within your range of movement. The quality of your awareness is more important than how far you can move. Repeat a few times, then reverse the direction of the rotation. Do this on each side, then both sides at the same time.

Hugging Arms

Inhaling, extend both arms out in line with your shoulders, palms forward, keeping your shoulders relaxed (see figure 24a). Exhaling, draw both arms across your chest, crossing the arms and giving yourself a hug (see figure 24b). Continue opening and closing your arms in this way, allowing the rhythm to be set by the breath; you can alternate which arm is on top. As your arms open, feel how the chest opens when the shoulder blades draw toward one another at the back. When your arms cross, feel how the upper back broadens and opens. Allow the movement to gently massage the spine.

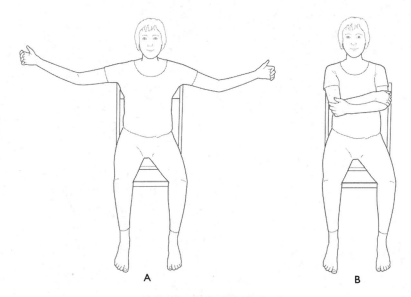

A   B

FIGURE 24: HUGGING ARMS

Taking Off a Top

Start with your arms hanging loosely by your sides. Following an in-breath, extend both arms in line with your shoulders, palms facing downward (see figure 25a), keeping the shoulders relaxed. Exhale and

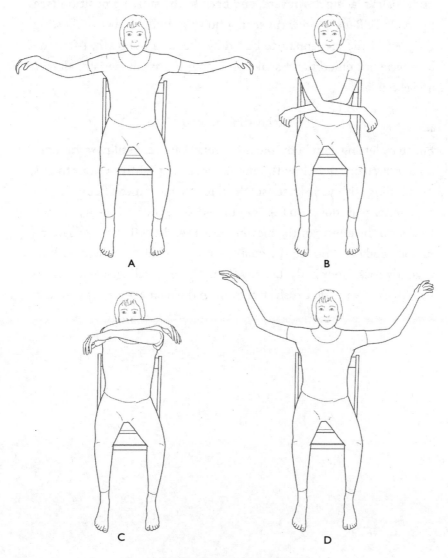

A   B

C   D

FIGURE 25: TAKING OFF A TOP

cross the arms in front of your body (see figure 25b). On the next inhalation, imagine you're peeling off a sweater by picking it up with both hands and raising your crossed arms up over your head (see figure 25c). On the exhalation, allow your arms to float down the sides of the body, palms facing downward, and back to the starting position (see figure 25d). Repeat a few times in a flowing rhythm, always allowing the pace of the movement to be led by the natural breath. After the last cycle, sit quietly and shake your fingers, hands, wrists, elbows, and shoulders.

Relaxation to End

Finish by letting your body and mind relax back into stillness. You can do this by sitting quietly with your hands resting lightly on your thighs, or standing with your knees soft and feet firmly on the floor. Or you may prefer to lie down on the floor or bed. Give yourself plenty of time to absorb the effects of the movements. Feel the different sensations in your body and notice the quality and movement of the breath as it gently rocks your body. Let any thoughts and feelings come and go, making sure you don't rush straight into the next activity of your day.

PART IV

Introducing Meditation

CHAPTER 9

What Is Meditation?

I want to ask you: In this whole world
What is the most profound
most wonderful thing?
Sit erect and meditate right to the end
As you meditate you'll find a clue
And everything will naturally become clear
Keep your concentration
don't miss your chance
After a while your mind will be pure
your wisdom right.
Then you won't have to fool yourself any more

RYOKAN, ZEN MASTER[1]

So far, this book has explored the quality of mindfulness, and although you may sense its value, mindfulness doesn't often come naturally. Our minds are usually full of chattering stories about the past and the future; our attention roams from one experience to another. Mindfulness needs to be consciously cultivated, and it takes discipline and commitment to gradually retrain how you relate to what you think and feel. That's where the systematic, regular practice of meditation comes in. People have practiced meditation for thousands of years, and they do so for many reasons; but as taught in this book, the aim of meditation is simply to develop mindfulness and kindness. The chapters in this section introduce meditation, offer advice on helpful attitudes toward meditation, and look at special issues for people meditating with chronic pain of one sort or another.

The following section, part 5, will explain how to establish your own meditation practice and will introduce three practices that are especially helpful for those working with pain, illness, fatigue, and stress. There is also some in-depth advice on how to work creatively with your thoughts and emotions.

MEDITATION

There are hundreds of meditations, including practices that calm the mind by focusing on an object such as the natural breath. Some involve contemplation of God, the Divine, or Reality, while others involve visualizing symbolic shapes and forms or cultivating loving-kindness. Often people have the idea that meditation means "not thinking," but some meditation practices utilize thought through directed contemplation, while others involve becoming aware of the thoughts themselves as they come and go without identifying so strongly with their content. Although meditation is commonly associated with the major spiritual traditions, especially Buddhism, in the West meditation has more recently been adapted to secular settings, including health care.

The meditation practices in this book have a simple structure and can be done by anyone regardless of their religious beliefs and the state of their physical health. They don't involve "mind control" or complicated visualizations; they are simply a training in becoming more aware of experience as it happens with a kindly, warm, and interested attitude. This brings choice and frees you from being a victim of impulses and habits.

You can do these practices sitting or lying down, and they can be practiced in almost any setting, including the hospital. When I was recovering from surgery a few years ago, I packed my CD player and did the three main meditations introduced in this book in part 5. It made a big difference to my mental and emotional experience, even when I was in severe pain, partially paralyzed, and bedridden.

Training in these ways brings an emotional stability that allows you to fully experience strong emotions while maintaining perspective on them, and with this comes wholeness and integration. Of course, most of us usually find it hard to do this, especially when dealing with intense pain or illness. Regular meditation using these methods can bring tremendous confidence, strength, and empathy within each meditation session and throughout the whole of your life.

MEDITATION IN WESTERN HEALTH CARE

Increasingly meditation is viewed as good medicine. It is used in many mainstream hospitals and clinics, especially in the United States, and extensive research demonstrates its effectiveness. Studies of people with chronic pain show that mindfulness reduces the level of pain they report and improves other medical and psychological symptoms.[2] Our own research at Breathworks shows improvement in every field we've measured: pain experience, quality of life, depression, the tendency to catastrophize, the ability to control and decrease one's experience of pain, and confidence in activity despite pain. The Breathworks program brings most people greater acceptance of their pain, improves their ability to maintain perspective, and increases awareness of beauty and kindness to themselves and others; it also brings a greater sense of choice, especially in response to unpleasant experiences.[3]

Mindfulness also helps people with conditions such as cancer, heart disease,[4] depression, anxiety, binge-eating disorders,[5] and hypertension (high blood pressure).[6] A recent study using brain imaging showed that meditation increased antibodies, suggesting it strengthens the immune system.[7] It also increases left-sided brain activity, which is associated with positive emotional states.

A 1995 report on alternative medicine for the National Institutes of Health that surveyed the data concluded that "meditation and similar forms of relaxation can lead to better health, higher quality of life, and lowered health–care costs . . . [by showing] how to live in an increasingly complex and stressful society while helping to preserve health in the process."[8]

MEDITATION AS TRAINING FOR LIFE

Meditation practice is not an end in itself; the aim is not simply to have "good meditations" but to learn to be more awake and kind so you can take these qualities into daily life. This can vastly improve your behavior and your relationships with others and make you a positive influence in the world. A friend of mine once described meditation as making her a safer person to be around. She's very serious about the effect she wants to have in the world, and she takes her meditation practice very seriously for this reason. Just as doctors take the Hippocratic oath of "doing no harm," so too can you take responsibility for your destructive emotions when they arise and try not to cause harm through blindly reacting to others.

Meditation training is often referred to as "practice" in the same way that a musician practices scales or an athlete trains his or her body. Not only does practice help you become a skilled meditator, it also allows you to become an emotionally positive human being whose life includes choice, initiative, kindness, and wisdom. The best way to tell if your meditation practice is effective is to look at how you're behaving *outside* meditation.

I often describe meditation as "the laboratory of self." You set aside a time that's free from interruptions, find a calm and peaceful place, settle into a physical posture that's relaxed yet alert, and close your eyes. When you do this you're calming the external senses and allowing your body to be still; it gives you the chance to slow down and turn your attention inward in a spirit of inquiry and receptivity.

You can then directly contact the heart and mind and discover what's really going on — just like a scientist looking through a microscope or a sculptor getting to know his or her raw material so that it can be shaped into a beautiful form.

THE BREATHWORKS APPROACH TO MEDITATION

The meditations introduced in this book have been chosen with care. These practices are easily accessible for those dealing with pain, illness, and stress, and they offer a balanced approach to developing awareness and kindness. All three complement one another and build on each other incrementally. Each practice will later be described in detail, but for now here's a brief overview of how they fit together.

Meditation 1: The Body Scan

The first practice I suggest you learn is the body scan (described in chapter 13), as this is a gentle way of learning to inhabit both the body and the moment. It's generally practiced lying down, and you can use the breath to accept areas of pain and tension and let go of resistance. The body scan is also a good practice for learning to pay attention to one thing at a time as you rest your awareness deeply within each part of the body in turn.

Meditation 2: Mindfulness of Breathing

Next, I suggest you move to the mindfulness of breathing (described in chapter 14), which is slightly subtler. It's widely practiced and has been popular for thousands of years, probably due to its simplicity and its profound benefits. Paying attention to the breath anchors your attention in the body, and this enables you to hold your experience within a spacious awareness — noticing thoughts, sensations, and emotions as they come and go. This awareness neither suppresses what's happening (for example, sensations of pain, illness, fatigue, or stress) nor does it overidentify with it.

Meditation 3: Kindly Awareness

In many respects, kindly awareness (described in chapter 15) is at the heart of the Breathworks approach to meditation. It builds on the connection with the body and the breath developed in the other practices, but broadens the field of your awareness to include a sense of empathic connection with others.

Three Doorways

The three practices offer slightly different routes to the shared aim of developing awareness and kindness. Imagine a large, airy house, at the center of which is a peaceful room perfumed with these beautiful qualities. To enter the room you can pass through one of three doorways of slightly different shapes and colors. The body-scan doorway is earthy and grounded; it's slightly below floor-level, so you have to step down to pass through it. This door requires a slow, observant pace that allows you to notice how your body feels. Meanwhile, the mindfulness-of-breathing doorway is painted sky blue and blows in the breeze, responding to the atmosphere inside and outside the room. The kindly-awareness door is deep red, and other people are passing through it beside you. It's impossible to go through this door without being aware of relatedness and interconnectedness, yet there's no sense of rushing.

"STOPPING" AND "SEEING"

Each of these practices includes the dimensions of "stopping" — calming or settling the mind — and "seeing," which brings insight into the nature of experience itself, enabling you to relate to life from a more fluid, broad, and stable perspective.[9]

Stopping or Calming Down

The skills of attention, focus, and concentration are the foundation of meditation. This process of calming down is sometimes described as "stopping" because you are learning to prevent the mind's hapless wandering and to become still and more awake. It's hard to reflect on your circumstances and to learn new ways of responding if the mind roams like a wild animal. So the first step is to tame it through simple exercises in paying attention to one thing at a time: for example, to parts of the body in the body scan, to counting the breath in the mindfulness of breathing, or to resting your attention on pleasant and unpleasant sensations in the kindly awareness practice. If you can focus your mental and emotional energies into a sharp beam of awareness, you will emerge from a foggy and diffuse state to one that's bright and clear.

Seeing

The second skill is using this focused awareness to discern the true character of your experience. Sometimes this is described as "seeing" or "seeing into the nature of things." It means learning to directly perceive your moment-by-moment experience as a *process* instead of being caught up with the *content*. As I've already said, if you examine the experience that you call "pain," you'll discover that it's a flow of changing sensations and responses rather than a fixed or hard thing. When pain is perceived in this way, you can become interested in the quality of the sensations rather than the stories you tell yourself about them — which are often distorted through fear, anxiety, and despair.

This fluid, creative attitude can transform your experience of yourself and dramatically alter your perceptions of other people and the world around you. You feel part of the flow of life rather than separated and isolated; you stop identifying with the choppy waves on the surface of the ocean whipped up by passing storms. Your awareness drops down into the depths, and you view the churning waves from the calm and stable perspective of the ocean itself. The experience is the same, yet somehow you see it in an entirely new way.

This suggests another important dimension of seeing. Not only do you relate to your own experience from a broader and deeper perspective, but also meditation becomes training in compassion and interconnectedness. As you become intimate with the nuances of your experience, you also explore what it means to be human. Whatever your experience, you can be sure that someone else is going through something similar at this very moment. Although the particulars of your own experience are unique, the human condition is common to all. We all want to be happy and to avoid suffering; we're all trying to avoid the unpleasant and to prolong the pleasant; we know the sense of rightness that arises when we relax into a sense of harmony with the way things are.

The Buddhist teacher Pema Chödrön says: "When you're happy, think of others; when you're in pain, think of others."[10] Anything you experience can be a moment of connection and empathy. The more you turn toward your experience in meditation and really get to know yourself with kindness and clarity, the more you can know humanity. When you journey within with honesty and courage, it can seem as if you sink through the particulars of your personal experience and touch the universal. Through meditation practice not only do you transform your relationship to illness and pain, you also become a more considerate and benevolent force for good in the world.

CHAPTER 10

Helpful Attitudes

Enough. These few words are enough.
If not these words, this breath.
If not this breath, this sitting here.
This opening to the life
we have refused
again and again
until now.
Until now.

DAVID WHYTE[1]

Meditation is an opportunity but also a challenge. I've already described how meditation can help, but sometimes it can also feel like a struggle. Your thoughts and feelings seem to have a life of their own, and you may feel that your meditation is continually hijacked by compulsive habits of thinking and disturbing emotions. If you live with pain and illness, you can feel that your experience of the body stubbornly gets in the way of the tranquility for which you yearn. Before you know it, you're assailed by doubt and despondency and start thinking, *I can't meditate.* Meditation can become yet another thing that you feel you've failed at, in a life that already contains many difficulties.

In this chapter I want to suggest a more helpful attitude toward meditation that has nothing to do with failure and success. I'll also offer simple tips on working with common difficulties.

BECOMING A HUMAN BEING, NOT A HUMAN DOING

The attitude I have in mind was wonderfully described by Sheila:

❋ **SHEILA**

In the space of two years I've had a brain tumor, a spinal tumor, osteo-porosis, and degenerative lung disease, and gone from working full time in a busy job and having many hobbies to being mostly housebound and taking large doses of morphine to manage the pain. But the hardest thing is the immense fatigue the brain tumor causes.

I've always been driven, moving at speed from one task to another. The jobs list I set for myself each day is fearsome and, I'm realizing, com-pletely unrealistic for somebody like me who's ill. I struggle through a few things on my list and get ever more frustrated at what I haven't achieved. I was expecting the Breathworks course just to help me with pain control, but it's changing my whole way of looking at life. I'm dis-covering that I need to develop other ways of living and to look at the qualities that make life worthwhile, not the number of tasks I complete.

This week my tutor asked me to develop more spaciousness around activities. I'm learning that it's possible to feel loved and supported for who I AM, not what I can DO. I'm learning for the first time in my life that I am a *human being* and not a *human doing!*

Becoming a "human being" rather than a "human doing" is a wonderful way of describing the spaciousness you can contact through meditation. Even though Sheila has severe physical difficulties, she's facing her limitations and tendencies honestly and learning a different way to be.

You might get away with rushing from one thing to the next when you're fit and healthy, but it's a recipe for self-destruction when the body is ill or tired. Even if you take up meditation, one danger (which Sheila has avoided, but many people fall into) is to transfer the habits of "doing" to meditation itself. Meditation becomes another thing to get right and succeed at, and it's easy to think that a successful meditation should be pleasurable, even blissful. For those of us with chronic pain, it can become another way of trying to escape our condition. But meditation isn't about manipulating life to get it on your own terms or to get rid of painful experiences, so how can we change these deep-seated habits and attitudes that are so familiar we often don't realize we have them?

Mindfulness helps in changing unhelpful habits because it requires engagement with experience in the moment, just as it is. This experience includes whatever primary suffering you have, whether pain in the body, fatigue, or whatever causes you stress and anxiety. Softening your response to the experience can dramatically alter it for the better — sometimes lessening pain, for example. But you need to make peace with any residual pain or difficulty by resting in the experience of the moment, whatever it contains, and meditation is the space in which you can learn to do so.

If you don't notice the reflex to resist any experience that you don't like, you may try to block out your pain by compulsively chasing distractions, or you might feel overwhelmed, as if you're drowning in difficulties. Either way, you end up living reactively rather than creatively, and moments, days, months, and years go by in a dense thicket of suffering.

Courageously bearing with the whole of your experience in meditation, you learn how to live *with* your circumstances rather than *against* them. If you bring this attitude to your meditation, gradually you will emerge from a state of restlessness and distraction into one of honesty, initiative, and choice. You can contact a sense of inner space and stability deep in the body that's unshakable, no matter what's happening. Bamboo is a traditional symbol of this kind of stability and flexibility. Its stalk bends with the wind, but it never snaps, and it remains rooted in the earth — strong, yet pliable and responsive.

If you can learn in meditation to include any painful sensations present within your awareness, you'll also discover they're just one aspect of the flow of life. You see more deeply into life and how things are for all of us. Imagine your life is a bottle of murky water continually shaken, so the water is always cloudy. When you meditate, you let the water settle, and the sediment naturally sinks to the bottom, leaving the water clear and still. Just as water naturally settles if it isn't shaken, you may find that your mind and heart want to settle if you give them a chance. It can be a surprising relief to stop rushing about, resisting and avoiding being with yourself, and instead to rest quietly in the moment. This brings stability and strength, even if your experience includes pain or difficulty.

The most beautiful way I know to describe the meditative state is *equanimity*. This is the central training of mindfulness meditation. You cultivate a state of body, heart, and mind that's kindly and sensitive, yet vibrantly alive. The mind will probably wander into thoughts of one sort or another, within meditation and within daily life — that's its nature — but mindfulness means noticing this and coming back to equanimity and rest, over and over again.

MEDITATION REFLECTION

Imagine a still lake at night whose surface perfectly reflects a full moon. The water is completely undisturbed, and so is the moon's reflection. A clear mind in meditation is like the clear water of the lake. A mirrorlike mind is wise and deep. It doesn't distort events and experiences, it reflects them back just as they are, without disturbance or corruption.

THREE KEY QUALITIES: INTENTION, ATTENTION, AND INTEREST

Intention

When I attended a workshop with Jon Kabat-Zinn a few years ago, he started by getting us to sit quietly and ask ourselves the question, "Why am I here?" We had all paid money, and some people traveled halfway across the world to attend—but asking that question helped us connect more consciously with our purpose. Without that we would perhaps have drifted through the event.

The same applies in each session of meditation. Once you're settled in your posture, it helps to engage consciously with your purpose. This helps you stay focused and engaged with the practice. You can ask, "Why am I meditating? What do I hope to gain from this session? Why do I want to be more aware?" The answers probably relate to your core motivations and deepest values. For example, if you're living with pain, then your intention might be to stop running away from it and to cultivate a broad, stable awareness that enables you to bring choice into situations usually driven by reactions and habits.

Your way of engaging with your purpose might be nonverbal. Often when I meditate a moment comes when I feel I've "landed," and suddenly I feel engaged with and interested in my experience. It seems that a sort of physical memory of meditation is evoked after I've been sitting for a while, and once more I'm in contact with my deeper motivations and the benefit I've received from meditation. This only happens if I remember to be kindly, then the memory emerges naturally into my experience.

Attention

If your intention is the context for your meditation, the task within each session is to be clearly aware of what's happening without pushing away those aspects of experience that you dislike and clinging to those you do like. So while you intend a particular outcome, the aim is also to be open to your experience as it is. This is sometimes called "the paradox of change."[2]

The Paradox of Change

If your goal is to respond to pain with more kindness and choice, you're unlikely to achieve this by straining for an outcome in a way that overrides how you actually feel. You're more likely to reach this goal if you take responsibility right now for your mental and emotional states. Finding a creative response in the present sets up positive conditions for the next moment. If you continually find such responses, peace will arise naturally. In other words, the only way to reach your future goals is to live fully and creatively in the present. The best way to get from A to B is really to be at A.

An experience of mine illustrates this. One morning when I sat down to meditate, I was experiencing back and neck pain and feeling nauseous. I felt reluctant to engage with meditation, but I knew that it would do me good to settle into my experience. After sitting for a while I realized I wanted the meditation to make me feel better and that the tension in my body came from willing this outcome. I saw that I wasn't being with my experience in a gentle way, so I settled my awareness in my body, and I had a lovely sense of coming to rest. The longing for my experience to be different fell away. When the meditation session ended I was able to move quietly back into activities, taking the day one moment at a time. Letting go of expectations in the meditation session meant that kindly, mindful awareness entered my day, and I could engage with activities without feeling anxious.

Being and Doing, and Balanced Effort

A similar paradox concerns effort and noneffort, or "being and doing." As Sheila wrote, through practicing meditation and mindfulness you learn to become a human being, not a human doing. But surely some effort is involved? You can't just lie down, give up all effort, and just be. Those of us living with painful bodies would probably never get up again!

Deciding to meditate, establishing your posture, and turning your attention to your object of meditation, such as the body and the breath, all involve effort. But this effort is in the service of being present to your experience. You could describe it as doing for the sake of being.

The effort we need in meditation is sensitive and receptive, like the effort of listening rather than the effort of shouting.

Balanced effort avoids both forceful striving and passivity. It's the effort of an eagle that hovers, perfectly balanced and poised on thermal currents, yet fully alert. It's the effort needed to cut a freshly baked loaf with a sharp knife: if you press too hard, the loaf will squash and flatten, but if you don't press hard enough, you can't slice it. You can experiment with balanced effort when opening doors or driving a car. What's the right amount of effort to apply so you don't forcefully grab the doorknob or the steering wheel, but open the door with effortless grace or hold the wheel with a light responsive touch? Similarly, in meditation you need to make enough effort to stay engaged with the practice, but you also need to be receptive to your experience.

The paradoxes of making effort in the service of effortlessness and of doing in the service of being suggest the magic of mindfulness. Often shining the light of awareness onto an experience is all you need to do to effect change. If you're clear about your intention and values, then as soon as you notice what's happening, your natural emotional and mental response will be shaped by those intentions.

Intention and Attention

In other words, if you're clear about your *intention* and values, and also pay *attention* to your experience in each moment, the future naturally takes care of itself. For example, if you notice that you're preoccupied with anxious thoughts, take a moment to check the underlying state producing these thoughts. Perhaps you notice that you feel contracted, stuck, and passive. The art of mindfulness is to notice those states without automatically reacting to them.

When you notice the gap between your intention, say, to live with initiative and choice and your experience of feeling stuck and passive, your experience naturally softens, provided you don't judge yourself harshly. As soon as you shine the light of awareness onto your experience, you can come to rest in the present moment and reconnect with the larger perspective of your intention to move toward freedom.

Interest

Attention and intention both depend on another quality: interest. You'll find it impossible to pay attention if you're more interested in your fantasies and distractions than your object of meditation, and hours of meditation can pass as the mind wanders aimlessly from one thought to another.

Interest in the Meditation Object

It isn't surprising that many of us find it difficult to maintain interest in something so subtle as the breath or the body's sensations, given the time we spend being stimulated by external interests such as watching TV, reading, surfing the Internet, talking, going to the movies, shopping, and so on. There's nothing wrong with these things in themselves, but the barrage of input can make it hard to calm down enough to be sensitive to inner experience. So, an important question when you're learning to meditate is, "How do I become interested in the object of meditation?"

In some meditation sessions you might feel that you never reach a settled state, and you may sometimes overcompensate and focus too tightly, as if your mind is crushing the object of meditation. If these things happen, don't worry. However much the mind wanders you can always have moments of *noticing* that your interest is drawn elsewhere. When you remember to come back to the breath, the body, or the current stage of the kindly awareness practice, you engage your interest and attention, if only for a moment. For most of us, the process of catching the mind and calling it back is how meditation usually proceeds. Figure 26 shows this process in a time line of a meditation session.[3]

Sometimes it seems impossible to stay with the object of meditation at all—perhaps you feel overwhelmed by your mental, emotional, or

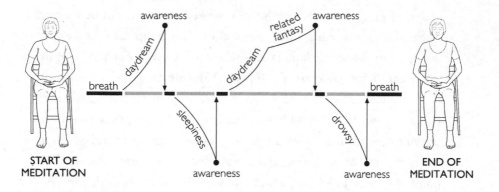

Typical experience through the duration of a meditation session. The horizontal line represents the object of awareness, e.g., the breath. The bolder sections represent periods of maintaining awareness of the breath, when you call the mind back from wandering.

FIGURE 26: A MEDITATION SESSION

physical experience. At such times, it's easy to get into an exhausting battle with yourself. Instead of calling the mind back with gentleness, the moment you notice a distraction, you yank the mind back to the meditation object before immediately bouncing off into distraction again. This clearly won't be a helpful way to meditate, and sometimes it's better to work *with* the power of the mind rather than to oppose it.

Patience Tames the Wild Horse

Our usual efforts to drag the mind back to its object of concentration are like the methods of a horse trainer who breaks in a wild horse by violently yanking on the bit and bridle until the animal is bullied into submission. That works in a way, but the tamed horse will probably be sullen and suspicious. If you do something similar in meditation, you may end up with a sullen and suspicious mind that moodily lurks around the breath, rather than a relaxed and confident one that enjoys the experience of breathing.

A gentler approach is wonderfully evoked in an account by Monty Roberts, a "horse whisperer" — someone who trains wild horses by being attuned to their language — who tamed a wild mustang colt in the Great Plains of America's Midwest.[4] The mustang was strong, and if Monty had used force he'd have had an impossible battle. Instead, he let it run and followed behind on his own horse, going wherever the mustang went on a wild ride that lasted more than a day. Eventually the mustang slowed and acknowledged his presence. At that point Monty stopped his pursuit and went in the other direction; the mustang followed out of curiosity with no force from Monty. Within thirty-six hours, he had earned the horse's trust, and within hours a rider was on its back.

This is a wonderful analogy for working with the mind if it behaves like a wild mustang. If you try to force it to stop, it will buck and kick, and you'll be exhausted by the struggle. But if you let the mind roam, it will settle down of its own accord. It only struggles because you oppose it. If you're patient, eventually the mind will become curious about the object of meditation just as the mustang did when it turned to follow the rider.

My colleague Sona describes how he once used this approach in the kindly awareness practice. Instead of feeling a kind connection with the people he was bringing to mind, he just felt irritable! Rather than simply trying to stop feeling irritated and to go back to what he thought he ought to be doing, he allowed the irritation to become part of his experience as he breathed in and out. He just sat: breathing in with irritation and breathing out with irritation, without judging himself for failing at the practice. Quickly, the irritation settled, and he felt a more genuine connection with others. Initially, the irritation had his interest rather than the kindly awareness practice. By accepting this, the tension that produced it gently dissolved, and his underlying intention to develop kindliness came to the fore.

Another time Sona was supposedly doing a session of the mindfulness of breathing, but instead he was in fact fantasizing about sailing in Sweden, where he used to live. Realizing he was more interested in the sailing fantasy than the breath, he decided to introduce the mindfulness of breathing *into* his sailing fantasy. He imagined breathing in and breathing out as he sailed along. Soon he lost interest in the fantasy and was able to gently guide his interest back to the breath and body.

Interest isn't something you can force. You need to coax and encourage the mind to make a connection with the object of concentration, perhaps noticing where the mind's interest lies at present and using that as a bridge to the meditation. You need the sensitivity of a horse whisperer as you get to know how your mind works, what interests it, and how it can be guided toward peace. Another way of describing this is developing a "wise perseverance" in reminding yourself to be aware.[5]

OTHER GENERAL TIPS FOR MEDITATION

Planting Seeds

It's easy to become overly concerned with immediate results and to give up when they don't come, so it helps to take a long-term view of meditation practice. Our lives are affected by many things over which we have little control. A relative dies, and you're plunged into grief; a deadline at work creates stress, and you can't settle in meditation. Perhaps you get the flu, so you can't meditate for a few days, and when you get back to it, the momentum has been lost. Such things are normal parts of life, but somehow you need to ride the ups and downs without giving up.

Whenever you meditate, you plant seeds. When a farmer does this, he has faith that crops will sprout and grow. You need faith that over time meditation will bring more awareness and initiative. Jon Kabat-Zinn says of mindfulness practice, "You don't have to like it; you just have to do it."[6] That's good advice. If you get caught up in assessing whether an individual session has been good or bad, then you may lose the bigger perspective. Regardless of how you might feel, you need to practice day after day, planting the seeds of mindfulness. If I want to assess the benefits of my practice, I find it helpful to look back over six months or more. With that perspective I can see if I'm more aware and happy, even though there may have been many ups and downs along the way.

Setting Up Helpful Conditions

Sona often says that if you find meditation difficult and are plagued by distraction you probably need to look at your whole life, not just your meditation. The quality of your meditation will be affected by the activities of your day. When you spend your whole day rushing madly about, you'll probably find it hard to engage with meditation in the evening. If you roll out of bed in the morning and try to meditate right away without properly waking up, you may well find your meditation sluggish and sleepy. When you're harsh and unkind to yourself and others during the day, it might feel impossible to engage with the kindly awareness practice. If you take medication in the mornings without having breakfast, you may feel nauseous and fuzzy-headed.

These things may seem obvious when you read them here, but it's surprising how little attention even experienced meditators pay to creating conducive conditions for mindfulness. If you can pace your activities throughout the day, be as fit and as mobile as possible, eat and sleep as well as possible, then it will be easier to meditate (see chapter 17 for more on how your daily activities can support your meditation practice).

Beginner's Mind

One of the great pitfalls in meditation is having expectations based on past experience. For example, you might have found it helpful to rest your awareness on the sensations in the abdomen in the mindfulness of breathing practice yesterday. Without really thinking about it, you do the same thing today, but this time it feels a bit wooden and dull. Maybe it would have helped to start by checking how you feel, which might have led you to try resting the awareness higher in the body.

If you maintain the freshness and wonder of a beginner in every session, even if you've been meditating for decades, your practice will stay creative and interesting. The Zen Buddhist tradition has a delightful phrase for this fresh and innocent awareness: *beginner's mind*—and that attitude also keeps you humble and ready to learn. As the Zen teacher Shunryu Suzuki once said, "In the beginner's mind there are many possibilities, but in the expert's there are few."[7]

An Attitude of Play

Related to beginner's mind is bringing a sense of play and adventure to meditation. The practices in this book have a definite structure, but you can still be creative in your approach and responsive to your experience. If you find things getting tight, you can expand your focus and open up to lighter, more subtle experiences. Should you find your thoughts wandering, perhaps you need to ground your awareness by focusing it low in the body. You can make adjustments like these with a light, playful attitude rather than judging whether you're getting it right. No one gets meditation "right" all the time, but people who get on well with the practice treat it as an adventure in which they learn new things about the mind, the heart, the body, and the world.

It can also help to let go of structure altogether and see what happens. Sometimes I use the last few minutes of a meditation to see where my heart and mind take me—I just let them roam. It's important not to drift about for the whole session, so experiment with this sort of approach in a spirit of adventure and curiosity for just short periods of time.

CHAPTER 11

Meditating with Pain

I said what about my eyes?
"Keep them on the road."
I said what about my passion?
"Keep it burning."
I said what about my heart?
"Tell me what you hold inside it."
I said pain and sorrow.
He said:
"Stay with it."

RUMI[1]

WORKING WITH INTENSE PHYSICAL PAIN
OR DISCOMFORT

For many reading this book, the main challenge in meditation will be the painful sensations in your body. If this pain is chronic it will probably persist, no matter how effectively you work with your thoughts and emotions. The issue then is how to accept this unpleasantness without reacting to it.

If you find this prospect difficult, you are not alone! But gently facing pain in meditation, rather than remaining trapped in cycles of avoidance and unawareness and feeling overwhelmed, is a heroic act. Each moment of awareness is one of being true to your experience and taking a step toward living a fulfilling and creative life.

Awareness Is Not Endurance

In meditating with pain, *awareness* is not the same as *endurance*. Sometimes people think that being able to sit with pain means gritting their teeth stoically. But if your attitude is one of willful striving, you're bound to create tension, resistance, and stress, and this won't be helpful in the long run. Simple things can be done to help make the experience of meditating as comfortable as possible.

Take Time over Posture

I always encourage people to spend as much time as they need in attending to their posture. Only you can know what posture is most comfortable. You need to discover this through trial and error, and it may change over time. Chapter 12 includes helpful principles that you can use as a guide.

When I first started meditating I tried to sit cross-legged on the floor because I was foolishly trying to be a "good" meditator. This caused me a lot of extra pain, but I persevered, thinking I was being brave and strong. Eventually I started sitting in a chair, which was much easier on my back but increased my neck pain. For some years I tried chairs of different heights and various ways to support my hands in my lap. At other times I tried meditating while lying down, but often this led me to feel sluggish and sleepy. More recently I've knelt on a couple of yoga blocks with an inflatable stability cushion on top (see figure 27 and appendix 3). These days it seems to be a good posture for my body: it creates a neutral angle in the pelvis and helps my shoulders and neck

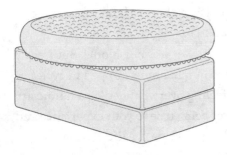

FIGURE 27: YOGA BLOCKS
WITH CUSHION

feel more aligned with the vertical axis running from the pelvis up my spine. The air cushion gives flexibility and balance throughout my spine.

I always have pain, but I think this posture is the best I can do for now. The process of trial and error that led me to this posture is likely to continue. A time will probably come when I can no longer kneel on the floor, and I'll have to engage creatively with other possibilities.

Length of Meditation Sessions

For some of us, sitting still for any length of time increases pain and tension, so you'll need to explore how long you can hold a certain posture. There's no benefit in sitting still for a long time if that increases your pain. On the other hand, like all meditators, people with pain are prone to restless and wriggly states of mind, and we can use our pain as an excuse to fidget. Sometimes remaining still can help settle the mind. The art of meditation includes distinguishing between the pain you need to listen to and the pain that comes from restlessness.

If your condition makes it difficult to remain still, you can either meditate for shorter periods or adjust your posture during a session. It's *your* body and mind, so find out what works for you. It's quite possible to lie down some time into a session without interrupting your focus and engagement. Should you need to stand and stretch, you can do so quietly and then sit down again. If you're meditating with others you'll need to move as quietly and mindfully as possible to avoid disturbing them, but taking that extra care can add to your awareness rather than interrupt it.

ATTITUDES TOWARD PAIN AND MEDITATION

I want to explore four main aspects of the attitudes that can help make meditation enjoyable and sustainable when meditating with pain.

Overcoming Resistance

The first hurdle is actually getting down to meditation. Even after meditating for twenty years I almost always have to overcome resistance — and I'm not alone. This tendency is especially pronounced if you're living with pain. When you meditate you turn toward your experience in an honest and open way, including your pain. That takes courage, but often I don't feel so brave, and when I contemplate meditating, suddenly I find many other things that need doing instead. *I'll make that phone call, I'll have another cup of tea, I'll check my e-mails.* Alternatively, I may think, *I can't bear to sit with myself and my pain — I'm too tired.* Then I roll over in bed and go back to sleep.

But I always regret it when I give in to the resistance, and I always feel better when I find the energy and courage to meditate. Even if I struggle in a particular session, I still end up feeling more honest and aware, which leads to more confidence and stability as I learn to be with my pain in a clear way. It's important to persevere and to recognize resistance rather than to be ruled by it.

Examining Your Agenda

Even when you've got down to meditating, attitudes still affect the practice, and it's important to investigate them. Most of us living with pain or illness long for our pain to go away, and you'll probably bring this desire with you when you start to practice meditation and mindfulness. No matter how much you think you've accepted your pain, many of us retain a secret hope that meditation will reduce or even eliminate it. On the face of it, this is entirely reasonable, but for people with intractable pain, mindfulness means coming to terms at the deepest level with the aspects of pain you can't avoid and making peace with the situation.

When I first encountered meditation in my midtwenties, I definitely brought an escapist agenda to my practice. I had intolerable pain, and I wasn't coping well; I wanted to escape my body and dwell in states of calm and bliss, and I hoped meditation would be a quick fix. That fantasy was understandable if you consider the ideas that circulate about meditation. I'd read books on Buddhism and meditation — and selectively remembered certain parts. Most of the literature gives a rounded picture of the human condition and describes how meditation can help you to be more awake. But instead I focused on descriptions of people who achieved meditative states in which they no longer experienced their body or described having a heart and mind that were vast, clear, and boundless, or described the body becoming so spacious and diffuse that it was like having a body of light. *Fantastic,* I thought, *I want some of that.*

These descriptions of higher meditative states were very attractive, and each time I meditated, I strained to be magically transported to a pain-free, blissful state. I even became adept at generating similar states through willpower and fantasy. At this stage, I would gather my awareness in my head, away from my painful body or outside my body altogether, and for a time the pain would lessen and I would feel calm and joyful. But there was also a lot of strain, and as soon as the meditation ended, I crash-landed back in my body and felt worse than before I'd started.

Many of us who learn to meditate when living with pain are motivated by a similar wish to escape the experience of the body. Friends who are skilled at meditating and who also live with painful bodies have told me that they had experiences of strain and escapism in their early meditation sessions that were very like my own. One woman, Eileen, who has a great deal of pain, told me how her practice has finally become much deeper and quieter.

✳ EILEEN

My body is aging and stiffening. More and more, I see this as an advantage, as I simply can't be very active, and the frustrations just have to be faced and accepted. My life has greatly simplified this year, internally as well as externally. I am seeing more clearly how I've pushed against life! Relaxation is what I'm learning now, and I'm discovering how unrelaxed I am at a deep level. I'm meditating much more than ever before, but without pushing at it. Life is more painful, but more real, and therefore more rich.

Another friend suffers from a degenerative spinal condition that causes him a great deal of pain and stiffness. He describes the end of an escapist meditation session as "crash-landing back in hell," which was very confusing and unpleasant. All three of us have now moved on to the next phase: using meditation to dwell ever more deeply *within* the body and using the experience of pain to cultivate equanimity and peace with life as it is.

One of the wonderful things about meditation is that it seems to bring out one's native intelligence and wisdom. If you meditate with sincerity and bring an unrealistic agenda, you'll realize that something's not quite right. In my case it took many years to realize this, but eventually instead of trying to move away from my experience, I turned to face it. I began the journey of engaging with my body with awareness.

Understanding the Paradox of Pain

I've already discussed "the paradox of change" — the principle that the best way to get from A to B is to be fully present at A. The same principle applies in coming into relationship with painful physical sensations. Rather than trying to move *out* of the body in a vain attempt to escape pain, the answer seems to lie in moving toward it, going more and more deeply *into* the body. This might seem a bitter pill to swallow; it's certainly counterintuitive. It may sound as if I'm suggesting that day after day, your whole meditation experience will involve sitting with awareness of pain. Hardly an inspiring prospect! But what I'm actually suggesting goes far deeper than that. To a large extent my meditation practice consists of simply sitting with an experience that includes the discomfort and pain, noticing the thoughts and emotions that arise, and working with my reactions to avoid piling on secondary suffering. But there are also times when I become awake to my experience in a very accurate and refined way. I sense that my awareness sinks deeply into my body, which starts to feel diffuse and spacious. The sense of space and translucence that fills me comes not from going outside myself into space, but from sinking so far inside that space and light seem to arise from within.

As a metaphor for this experience, consider the image of a tapestry such as one you might see in a country mansion or château. From a distance, the tapestry depicts a complex scene that looks dense and solid, but as you come closer you realize it's made up of thousands of colored threads. If you looked into the weave of the threads with a microscope, you'd see millions of tiny spaces in between the threads. Through meditation, you develop this open, expansive perspective as you find the spaces in the weave of your experience and gently rest there.

These experiences of profound spaciousness are part of the world opened up by meditation. They are the states that I'd read about and been drawn to when I first learned to meditate, but then I made the mistake of trying to bypass my body to achieve them. Only by sitting *with* the pain can one access intense joy. I like to say that the open sky lies *beneath* the earth. Feeling supported by the earth, you can take your awareness so far inside the body that you come to a place of peace and calm.

Focusing the Mind with Pain

Strong experiences of pain can sometimes help in focusing the mind. If your experience is very pleasant, it's easy to slip into a fuzzy, soft-focus state and daydream your way through meditation. Intense pain gives an edge to experience that can strengthen meditation. It isn't easy to do this, but Stefan, an experienced meditator who lives with chronic pain, describes it well.

❈ **STEFAN**

If I can stay in the pain, I can use it to get to a deeper level of meditation. Pain often has a lot of energy and focus tied up with it, but the only way of getting into the deeper state of concentration is to have a strong base, and that involves working through your body. I can experience this as meditating out of the earth; that's how deep and strong your base should be. When I meditate in that way, I usually experience a state of equanimity afterward, and then my whole experience of life is completely different. It's warmer, softer, and there's a broader view that gives me the wisdom to deal with my experience. I can't always access these states, but those moments help me enormously.

PART V

Meditation Practice

CHAPTER 12

Setting Up for Meditation

Before you embark on a formal meditation practice, it's helpful to learn how to set up your posture and to find the right time and place for practice.

POSTURE

For many of us, the word *meditation* brings to mind the image of a person sitting cross-legged on the floor in a very upright and stable posture. It's true that sitting cross-legged can be a helpful meditation posture for someone who's physically fit and very flexible, but few Westerners, even those who are fit and strong, can actually sustain it for long.

The main criteria in finding a posture for meditation are that the body is subject to as little muscular strain as possible and that the posture supports an alert, but relaxed, state of mind. Bearing this in mind, there are no restrictions whatsoever on suitable postures. If you're dealing with ill health or chronic pain, it's important to adapt creatively, so I encourage you to throw out the rule book — *including* some of the advice on posture in other books on meditation if no account is taken of those with physical incapacity. Be sensitive to your body and experiment until you find a posture conducive to meditation. Bear in mind that what suits you best may change over time, as your body goes through the natural aging process and the ups and downs of any chronic health condition you have.

For some this could mean lying down to meditate; others may prefer sitting on a chair, and some will find it most comfortable to kneel or sit cross-legged on the floor. Sometimes you may need to alter your posture within a meditation session, especially if you have a condition in which the body requires regular movement. But if you do move, try to include that in your meditation, moving as mindfully as you can.

Of the three formal meditation practices introduced in this book, the body scan is generally done lying down, though this isn't essential. The mindfulness of breathing and kindly awareness practices are probably best carried out sitting upright on a chair or on the floor, if that's possible for you, to reduce the chance of sleepiness.

I've already given some specific advice on posture for people with chronic pain or disability in chapter 11, but here are some general principles and guidelines.

Lying Down

If you meditate while lying down, it helps to find a setting in which you'll be comfortable but as awake as possible. Bear in mind a phrase that Jon Kabat-Zinn uses to describe the state of mind and body you're developing in meditation, even when lying down. He calls it "falling awake"—which means you need to be alert, as well as relaxed.

It may be better to lie on a mat on the floor rather than on your bed because the bed is usually associated with sleep. But feel free to lie on your bed for meditation if that's the only place you're comfortable. It's also the best place if you have sleep problems and are doing the body scan to help you relax and ease the transition into sleep.

For more advice on lying-down postures, especially getting the right support for your head and legs, see chapter 8 (page 100). Allow your hands and arms to rest on the floor at the side of your body with the palms facing upward, or rest them lightly on the belly or the hips with the palms facing downward. If you have a tender back, make sure you have sufficient padding beneath you so that undue pressure won't build up during the meditation practice.

Sitting Down and Balancing the Pelvis

Whatever sitting posture you adopt — in a chair, kneeling on the floor, or sitting cross-legged — the key to finding a comfortable posture is the angle of your pelvis. The pelvis is like the base of a pylon; it anchors the whole upper body, and its angle affects the alignment of your spine, neck, and head (see figure 28).

Because modern Westerners spend so much time sitting in chairs and at desks, many of us find the pelvis has a tendency to roll backward, causing the lower spine to lose its natural curve. This leads to rounded shoulders and a tendency for the head to protrude in front of the spine, producing tension in the neck (see figure 29a). If you can find a posture in which the pelvis is balanced and erect, the spine will follow its natural, gentle S curve. This allows the head to rest lightly at the top of the spine, and the back of the neck to be long and relaxed,

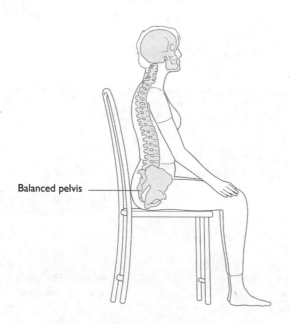

Balanced pelvis

FIGURE 28: BALANCING THE PELVIS

with the chin slightly tucked in. Through the base of the skull, a sense of openness naturally arises. A balanced pelvis also allows the legs to "fall outward" toward the floor and creates the least possible strain in the larger muscles of the thighs and hips.

A good way to find out if your pelvis is erect is to tip it backward and forward a few times, looking for the point of rest and balance in the middle. You can also try putting your hands under the fleshy cheeks of the buttocks while seated and feeling for the sitting bones — the bony tips deep within the buttocks that take the weight as the body sits upright. When the pelvis is balanced, most of the weight passes directly through these bones rather than via the fleshy pads at the back of the buttocks (see figure 29a) or the pubic area in front (see figure 29b).

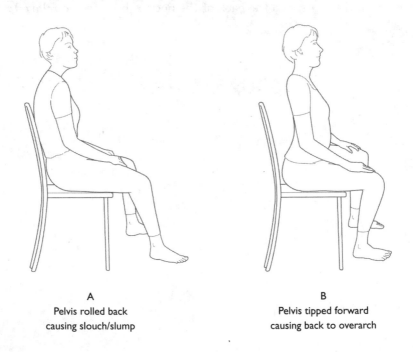

A
Pelvis rolled back
causing slouch/slump

B
Pelvis tipped forward
causing back to overarch

FIGURE 29: INCORRECT PELVIC POSITIONING

It's also important to rest your hands at the right height. You may want to support them on a cushion or have a blanket wrapped around you to help the shoulders remain open and broad instead of being drawn downward as the meditation progresses by the weight of the hands (see figures 30a and 30b).

Sitting on a Chair

If you decide to sit on a chair, it's best to choose one that's straight-backed, such as a dining chair. When your back is quite strong, it can help to sit forward on the chair, leaving the spine free to follow its natural curves and create a sense of openness in the chest that encourages alertness and emotional brightness. If your back is weak, place a cushion behind it to provide support while maintaining uprightness (see figure 31a).

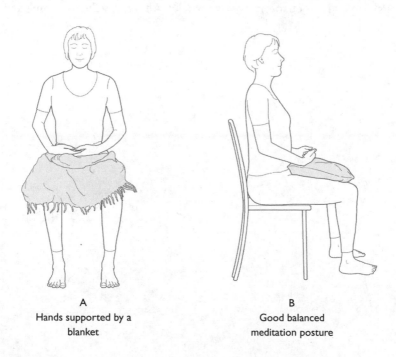

A
Hands supported by a
blanket

B
Good balanced
meditation posture

FIGURE 30: SUPPORTING THE ARMS

Make sure your feet are flat on the floor. If your legs don't quite reach the floor, place a cushion or pillow under your feet so they make firm and stable contact with the ground (see figure 31b).

Kneeling on the Floor

Some people with back problems actually find it's more comfortable to kneel on the floor to meditate than to sit on a chair. Often it's easier to adjust the pelvis so that it's balanced and erect when the thighs are at a less acute angle than the 90 degrees produced by sitting in a chair. On the other hand, kneeling on the floor is a bit harder on the knees and ankles, so work out what feels best for you.

If you do kneel, it's important to establish the right height and firmness. You may want to buy a meditation stool, some meditation cushions, an air cushion, or yoga blocks. Alternatively, use something

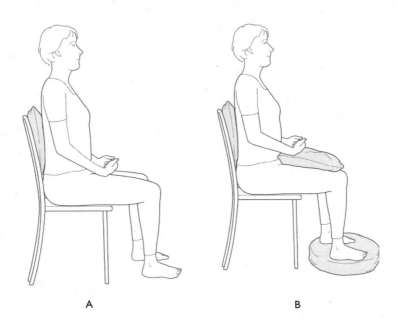

A   B

FIGURE 31: SITTING POSTURE ADJUSTMENTS

firm and stable, such as telephone books with a cushion on top for padding. Appendix 3 includes details of meditation materials.

The main thing is that your seat is neither too soft — which will make it unstable — nor too hard, as this will be uncomfortable. If it's too high, your pelvis tends to tip forward, overarching the lower back, and if it's too low, your pelvis may roll backward, rounding the back and shoulders. Both extremes create an unhelpful posture and may produce back pain, neck pain, and an overall sense of strain, so paying attention to the height of your seat is very important (see figure 32a).

If you experience strain in your ankles while kneeling, try supporting them with rolled-up socks (or similar) to take the strain off the ankle joints. Play around with what you have on hand, and see if you can get comfortable (see figure 32b).

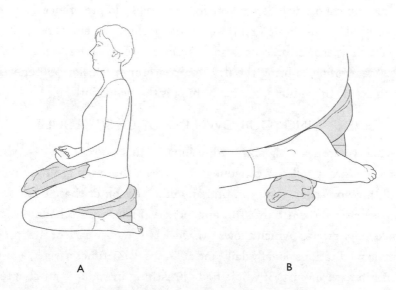

A   B

FIGURE 32: KNEELING POSTURE ADJUSTMENTS

Sitting Cross-Legged

The final option is to sit cross-legged on the floor, but because this requires quite a degree of flexibility in the hips, this particular posture is probably unsuitable for those dealing with chronic pain or chronic health problems. Unless you're very flexible, I suggest that sitting in a chair and kneeling on the floor are the two most desirable sitting meditation postures.

MEDITATING REGULARLY

Meditation can have a big effect, but you'll experience the benefits most fully if it becomes a regular part of your life. Be realistic about the length of time for which you can meditate. It's better to meditate regularly for manageable periods than to have intermittent attempts that are too long for you to sustain. Even ten minutes a day makes a difference.

For most people, finding time for meditation is a big challenge, and it helps to work out a regular slot to fit into your daily routine. The time you choose will depend on your lifestyle and preferences. Some people like to meditate first thing in the morning to help start the day off with a sense of presence and awareness; others prefer to meditate in the evening to bring the day to a peaceful conclusion. Whenever you decide to meditate, the main thing is that you do it!

CREATING YOUR OWN PRACTICE SCHEDULE

While you're learning the meditations in this book, I suggest you systematically follow a schedule that gives a thorough grounding in all three practices. (You can find an audio version of these exercises at soundstrue.com/burch.) In appendix 1, I suggest a schedule that takes eight weeks, which allows two weeks to practice each of the three main meditations, ideally daily and at least several times a week, along with breath inquiry 3: whole-body breathing introduced in chapter 7 (see pages 88–91). Once you've experienced all three meditations thoroughly, you can establish your own routine. You'll probably find some practices easier than others, but I suggest that you keep doing them all, alternating regularly, as they complement one another and offer a balanced approach to meditation and mindfulness.

Over time you may decide to do different practices at different times of the day, and you can then arrange them to help you manage your condition. For example, I do a sitting meditation practice in the morning for thirty to forty minutes, and after lunch I do a body scan lying down. I find this combination very helpful. The morning meditation enables me to tune in to myself and helps me to be positive and mindful throughout the day, while the body scan breaks up the day. Moving about, bending, and so on aggravates my spinal condition, so my pain usually increases as the day goes on. The body scan session creates a space in which I deeply rest my body and interrupt the buildup of tension. Although it means taking time out of whatever else I might be involved with, I reach the end of the day in a better state, physically, mentally, and emotionally.

TIMING SESSIONS

The mindfulness of breathing and the kindly awareness meditation practices are both divided into stages to provide structure to the meditations (see chapters 14 and 15). If you aren't using the led practices for guidance, you'll need to time the stages for yourself. Usually I place my watch on the floor in front of me and glance at it every now and then, which helps to create stages of roughly even length rather than spending fifteen minutes on the first stage and then rushing through the rest. You can also get a timer that clips onto your belt or clothing and vibrates at regular intervals to mark the stages (see appendix 3).

ENVIRONMENT

Another way of supporting a meditation practice is to create a pleasant and peaceful space for meditation. This could be as simple as having a quiet, tidy, and peaceful corner of your home. You may want to arrange a few flowers or burn some incense there to create a sense of beauty, or you might find it helpful to use an evocative natural object, such as a rock or a piece of driftwood. You could place photographs that evoke the peaceful state of mind that you're encouraging through meditation.

Creating this sort of space can be remarkably powerful. Sitting down amid mess and clutter won't help you develop inner calm and clarity, but sitting in a special space can bring a sense of ritual that encourages you to make the transition into a quieter, more contemplative state of mind. It also helps to turn off your phone and to let others in your house know that you would like to have this period of time undisturbed, if this is possible and appropriate.

As with all the suggestions in this chapter, the main thing is to think creatively about what will support your meditation and to create helpful conditions.

CHAPTER 13

The Body Scan

How surely gravity's law,
strong as an ocean current,
takes hold of even the strongest thing
and pulls it toward the heart of the world.
Each thing —
each stone, blossom, child — is held in place.
Only we, in our arrogance,
push out beyond what we belong to
for some empty freedom.
If we surrendered to earth's intelligence
we could rise up rooted, like trees . . .
This is what the things can teach us: to fall,
patiently to trust our heaviness.
Even a bird has to do that
before he can fly.

RAINER MARIA RILKE[1]

The body scan is a good place to start the journey of developing mindfulness through formal meditation. It's similar to Breath Inquiry 3 in chapter 7 (see pages 88–91), but now your awareness touches every part of the body in turn in a detailed and precise way. You can imagine you're washing your body, on the inside and the outside, with a flow of mindfulness.

This chapter includes a short body–awareness exercise (available as a downloaded audio file from soundstrue.com/burch) that gives a taste of the detailed awareness developed in the body scan. But I recommend you also use a longer fully guided version to get the full sense of the practice (see page 270). Then you can simply rest back and be guided through the meditation.

The practice is usually done lying down, if this is comfortable for you. If not, adopt any other posture that suits you. You may find your body temperature drops a little during the practice, so make sure you'll be warm enough, perhaps covering yourself with a blanket. (See chapter 12 for tips on posture.)

I first came across the body scan twenty years ago when I did it at the end of yoga classes; it was a revelation. The teacher invited me to feel into the different parts of my body, one by one, and all I had to do was lie there and let her gently and tenderly guide me deeper and deeper. It was such a relief to stop resisting the pain even if only for a few moments.

As I started to incorporate body-scan sessions into my daily life, deep habits of holding and tension gradually dissolved. The effects of the body scan are subtle, so I didn't experience a dramatic moment of release, but when I looked back after several months I saw how much more comfortable I was in my own skin. I now try to do the body scan every day after lunch, which helps me inhabit my body with a gentle awareness and guide it through the day with dignity. On days when I don't practice it, I often end up feeling tense and restless. I've been doing the body scan fairly regularly for more than twenty years now, and I have less tension, much greater awareness, and a vastly improved sense of well-being.

GROUNDING AWARENESS IN THE BODY

As we saw in chapter 7, it's important for those of us living with pain and illness to reinhabit our bodies because we tend to resist our physical experience and live in our head, only noticing the body when pain becomes unbearable. Breath awareness is an essential aid to gradually undoing these habits, and the body scan takes this more deeply by training you to ground your experience in the body. Rather than being dominated by thoughts, ideas, or fears *about* the body's sensations, you come into contact with the *actual sensations* you're experiencing. The effect is gentle and restful: you don't have to *do* anything at all, so you can soften any tension that has built up in reaction to your pain. It's a receptive and gentle practice — and a fantastic way to move back into the body with an attitude of invitation rather than demand. In addition, it can mysteriously and magically lead to profound levels of awareness.

The Zen teacher Shunryu Suzuki said that wisdom can arise gradually and imperceptibly, like walking through a fine mist and finding you're completely drenched without knowing how it happened.[2] Similarly, in the body scan you just do the practice, and by the end you feel quite different even though you may not have noticed exactly when your awareness changed.

THE PRACTICE

When you do the body scan you take your awareness to the different parts of the body, and as you rest your awareness in each place, simply notice what's happening, feeling that part of the body deeply, from within.

Sometimes people think that the instruction to be aware of the body means taking a bird's-eye view from the outside, but this isn't what's intended. If the instruction is to be aware of your big toe, for example, then the practice is to take the awareness right down inside the big toe and to be aware of whatever sensations present themselves. If you can't feel anything, it means being aware of the absence of sensations.

This awareness is nonjudgmental, so whether the sensations are intense or absent isn't important; the important thing is simply to be aware. If you notice tension and pain or discover an area that's numb, instead of thinking, *I'm going to try to change that,* just notice it with a gentle, kindly awareness. With consistent practice you'll develop increasingly subtle awareness of your body.

ROUTES AROUND THE BODY

There are many ways to do the body scan, and there are probably just as many opinions about the right way to do it! Some people leading it start at the feet and work up to the head; others begin at the head and work to the feet, while still others do one side of the body and then the other. I don't think there's any one right way, and often it comes down to the preference of the leader. However, different routes have subtly different effects, and it can be helpful to bear this in mind when deciding which route through the body you want to take in a particular session.

Head to Feet

For most of us awareness tends to be focused at the top of the body. The head is where we experience thinking, and most of the sense organs (eyes, ears, nose, and tongue) are in the head, so this is where awareness tends to reside. If you start the body scan at the head, then you're beginning at an area with the most awareness. If you move down through the body to end at the feet, you'll finish the session feeling much more grounded and quiet, so this is a particularly calming and quietening method. You're also more likely to feel sleepy at the end, so if you're doing the body scan last thing at night to calm yourself down for bed, this is a good way to do it.

Feet to Head

If you're already sleepy or lethargic at the beginning of the session, then you might prefer to start the body scan at the feet and end it at the head. Sometimes this can leave you feeling more alert and wakeful because, again, the head is the area normally associated with the active sense organs.

If You Have Pain to Start With

It can be hard to simply plunge your awareness into the body, and you may feel resistance to "going inside" if you have a lot of pain. You might find it easier to start the body scan at the head, which is probably where your awareness will be focused. Even if you feel dominated or overwhelmed by pain in the body, in most instances you'll probably find your awareness is still focused around the head because you're likely to be feeling a certain amount of anxiety, fear, and disturbed thoughts about the pain. If you start the session with the instruction, "Allow the awareness to rest in the feet," you'll probably find that difficult to follow because the feet can seem such a long way away. You may think, *I don't even know how to be aware of my feet—I can't even feel them!* So you might find it gentler to start the body scan at your head, where your awareness is already focused, and gradually connect with the body in the course of the practice as your awareness moves through it. You'll end up feeling deeply grounded and embodied.

EXERCISE: THE BODY SCAN

This short exercise will give you a taste of the body scan. (It is also available on audio at soundstrue.com/burch.) A more detailed led version is also available (see page 270).

SETTLING

Decide on your posture, loosen any tight clothing, and let your body settle onto the surface on which you're lying or sitting. Remember to cover yourself with a light blanket so you don't get cold. If you can, turn off the telephone and ask people to leave you undisturbed for the duration of the practice.

CONTACT WITH THE EARTH

As you sit or lie, bring your awareness to the points of contact between your body and the surface on which you're resting. If you're lying down, this is usually the back of the head, the shoulder blades, the upper and middle back, and the sacrum—the flat triangular bone at the base of the spine. Your elbows will probably be resting on the floor or bed, allowing your hands either to lie at the side of your body, palms upward, or to rest on your belly, hips, or ribs, palms downward. Choose whichever is most comfortable. If your legs are outstretched, let your feet fall out to the side.

Once you've felt these areas of contact, allow the body to sink down through them. Feel your body being supported by the earth without any effort or resistance from you; the earth is strong and easily able to take your weight.

BREATHING

Take your attention to your breathing. Spend a few moments resting your awareness on the movement of the body as the breath flows in and out, particularly the rise and fall of the abdomen. Remember to rest your awareness on the breath in the back of your body as well as the front. Allow the body to soften, particularly on the out-breath, and simply be aware of the body's sensations. Don't worry if you notice tension.

THE SCAN

Choose whether to start the body scan at your head or feet. It doesn't matter which way you do it; just see what feels right for you.

STARTING AT THE HEAD

Become aware of your head sinking down onto the pillow and allow it to feel heavier still, letting go of any strain to hold it up. Notice what happens at the base of your skull, where you might feel a sense of release and softening.

Allow your awareness to sweep the face and notice any sensations in the forehead, the cheeks, the mouth, and the jaw. Check if you're clenching your teeth and soften any holding. Let the jaw hang loose and soft, with the lips lightly touching if you're breathing through the nose; let the tongue be soft in the mouth.

Bring your awareness to the eyes and let them rest deep in the sockets behind the lids. Allow the broad expanse of skin between the eyebrows and the hairline to be smooth and soft.

STARTING AT THE FEET

If you begin with the feet, notice if they feel warm or cold. Allow your awareness to inhabit them, experiencing the sensations directly. If it's hard to keep your awareness in your feet, don't worry: each time you notice that your awareness has wandered, just bring it back to the feet. Take your awareness to the toes and move through them, one by one, becoming aware of any sensations you encounter without judgment. Let your awareness sweep through each foot, noticing any sensations on their soles or tops, and see how those sensations change, moment by moment.

THE REST OF THE BODY

Gradually take your awareness through your whole body, moving from one end to the other. Include the front and back, and remember your arms and hands. If you don't feel anything in a certain area, just notice that.

WORKING WITH TENSION

When you notice any pain or tension in a particular area, see if you can soften around it. You can do this using the breath: breathing in awareness to this area and letting go of resistance on the out-breath. Imagine the tension releasing into the earth. Just bringing awareness to your experience with a gentle attitude will encourage a natural sense of letting go.

CONCLUSION

Give yourself plenty of time to make the transition from the body scan. Be careful how you move your body after this period of stillness. If you've been lying down, roll gently onto one side and then come onto your hands and knees, if this is comfortable, before standing, keeping the head in line with the spine. Be careful to maintain the benefits of the body scan by avoiding awkward movements that strain your body unnecessarily.

THE TRANSFORMATIVE POWER OF AWARENESS

The reason you don't need to force change is that awareness is naturally transformative: when you become aware of tension, the natural response is to soften and let go of it. When you become aware of something painful, there's a longing for, and movement toward, release. A nurse at a pain clinic once said to me, "Relaxation is the natural state when you stop creating tension." I often remind myself of this phrase. The nurse's suggestion that spaciousness is natural while tension is something you create is a radical thought. Many of us think we need to *do* something in order to relax or experience peace when in fact we just need to stop putting effort into creating tension and strain.

LETTING GO, YIELDING, OR LETTING BE

Whether you do the body scan sitting or lying down, it can be lovely to let the weight of the body settle onto the earth. You get a sense that your body is held and supported by the whole planet beneath you: strong, stable, and more than able to support your weight. From the planet's point of view, you're as light as a feather.

As you let go of, or "yield," the weight of your body to the earth, it may become obvious how much unnecessary holding you do. While reading this page, notice whether you're allowing your weight to settle onto the surface on which you're resting. If you're sitting in a chair, notice if you're allowing yourself to rest back into the chair (without slouching), or whether you're holding your body against it with resistance and strain. Now notice what's happening in response to this awareness. If you noticed holding, have you also experienced a natural response of letting go, or yielding? This is the quality of awareness cultivated during the body scan. As you notice tension or holding, it's natural to soften and let go. You may experience tension arising again and again with the passing moments, so you let go, again and again. You can do this over and over without worrying about success or failure.

Allowing resistance to soften as you take your awareness through the body can be a huge relief, especially if you have chronic pain. Fear of the pain and the desire to avoid it mean you disconnect with your actual experience as it's felt in the body. The layers of avoidance take you further and further away from your immediate experience and bring secondary suffering. The body scan creates conditions that enable you to gradually move toward the pain with a kindly, gentle awareness.

I've already spoken of *letting go, letting be,* and *yielding,* and each term has slightly different connotations. Some people find "letting go" too active a phrase, while others consider "letting be" too passive. In different ways, these words attempt to evoke the quality of awareness that comes through the body scan, in which you feel what it's like to inhabit the body fully, with as little resistance and holding as possible.

❋ JAMES

I find the body scan very soothing because it softens everything. I really like inhabiting my shoulders because I habitually hold a lot of tension there, so I cut off and look at them from the outside. But if I can take my awareness right inside my shoulders, I can sink into them and give them a massage with the gentle movement of the breath. When I manage to stay with this kind of awareness, my tension and holding dissolve through my whole body and sink down into the earth; it's an amazing feeling. I also feel I'm giving my body the best possible chance of healing and resting.

USING THE BREATH

As we saw in chapter 7, the breath can be a powerful support in the body scan. When you come to each part of the body, you can imagine the breath entering it on the in-breath, and you can yield or let go down toward the earth on the out-breath. This can become a habit that helps in daily life. Old habits of holding and resistance may gradually be replaced by the helpful habit of breathing into an area of pain or discomfort and letting go on the out-breath. You can do this in any situation—standing in long lines, sitting on public transportation, wherever you are. Gradually this skill becomes second nature and a powerful ally in interrupting the habitual buildup of tension.

※ **BRENDA**

Brenda, a woman in her sixties, attended the Breathworks course to help her deal with allergies. One week she came to class and said she had invented a little chant that she said to herself throughout the day to help her use the breath to soften tension. On the in-breath she would say, "Hello" to her experience, whatever it was. On the out-breath she would say, "Let go." She said it really helped her deal with stress. Throughout the day she would softly recite to herself: "Hello; let go. Hello; let go. Hello; let go."

BODY AND MIND

The body scan is also a way to investigate directly the relationship between mind and body. Often people with pain or illness feel a split between the two, and it can be fascinating to investigate the relationship between them in your own experience and to look for a greater degree of harmony and rest. In addressing the responses to pain that create secondary suffering, trying to work on the mind alone isn't enough; you also need to work with the resistance in the body.

I see awareness as a continuum: body awareness is at the denser, grosser end of the spectrum, and awareness of thoughts and emotions is at the subtler, ephemeral end. But they are two aspects of the same thing; both involve awareness of the shifting complex of momentary experience. Sensations in the body give rise to thoughts and emotions, and these have echoes within the body. S. N. Goenka, a well-known Indian meditation teacher, said, "Every thought, every emotion, every mental action, is accompanied by a corresponding sensation within the body. Therefore, by observing the physical sensations you also observe the mind."[3]

The interconnectedness of the mind and body suggests that the body scan is much more than just a relaxation technique. Potentially, it's a profound awareness practice. Being honest about what's happening in your physical experience during the body scan in a direct, immediate, nonjudgmental way will also affect your mental and emotional states. Likewise, if you're in an agitated state, softening around physical tension and resistance may quiet the mind. It can be hard to work directly on the mind because it's slippery and elusive, but working with the more tangible sensations of the body offers a practical and effective means of calming down and even transforming your whole experience.

Those of us living with chronic pain and illness are bound to have some degree of mental and emotional tension and distress in addition to our physical pain or discomfort. Doing the body scan regularly will affect all these levels, not just the physical, because it undermines patterns of resistance, and it's a good starting point for formal meditation.

COMMON DIFFICULTIES WITH THE BODY SCAN

Falling Asleep

Falling asleep is common during the body scan. If you're tired, the body scan might enable you to experience some welcome rest, or the sleepiness could be an expression of resistance to becoming aware of your body. When introducing people to the body scan, I encourage them not to worry if they fall asleep, whatever the cause. Somehow, the practice still has an effect, as if the words of the instructor affect you subconsciously. The body scan can be helpful for sleeping problems. If it helps you to sleep during the day, it's likely that it will work at night as well. However, I suggest that in time you try to practice the body scan at a time of day when you're more likely to stay awake, as it will be more effective; gradually you can become more proficient at "falling awake" while remaining calm and quiet.

Wandering Thoughts

Wandering thoughts are very common, so there's no need to feel as if you've failed if you seem to be constantly distracted. Keep bringing the awareness back to the body over and over again, letting go of any worries about what you think should be happening.

Pain and Restlessness

See if you can remain aware of what's happening when you experience pain or feel restless, and make conscious choices in how you respond. Although most people prefer to do the body scan lying down, there are no rules. You can adopt any posture you want, choosing the one that's most likely to be comfortable. If you can't stay in the same position for the duration of the practice, by all means move. When I teach the body scan in classes, I always encourage people to move if they find their pain intensifies through being in one position, and often they like to roll onto their side part of the way through. Sometimes I do the body scan lying on my back, sometimes on my front, and sometimes on my side. If I feel the need to move, I carefully change position during the practice, which helps prevent pain from building up through pressure.

Do whatever you need to feel comfortable; the practice will be more beneficial if you don't have to fight feelings of pain or discomfort. Often it's easier to soften toward a dull ache than a stabbing or shooting pain; you are the best judge of that. If pain disturbs you, notice if you're holding your breath. Practicing optimal full-body breathing can help (see chapter 7).

❊ CHARLOTTE

I found the body scan difficult at first because I thought I shouldn't move at all, which was like torture. Now I use my imagination and do little movements, like gently moving my hips. I also visualize pleasant images or comforting things, like imagining I'm doing the body scan lying in a field under some beautiful trees or gliding on the top of Victoria Falls or lying in the arms of someone who's taking my weight and comforting me.

Sometimes the body is restless simply because the mind is agitated. By letting the body gradually settle onto the earth and remain quiet and still, the mind also quietens. It can be interesting to investigate whether a desire to move during the practice is caused by genuine pain — when moving would help — or by emotional restlessness — when staying still would be more useful. The main thing is to choose to move, without moving around compulsively. Try playing around with this distinction in different sessions of the body scan to see if you can be more in tune with what you need to do to bring about greater overall calm and ease.

Panic or Feeling Fearful

This is common if you are unaccustomed to being still and quiet. The feeling of panic or anxiety can be unpleasant, but it soon passes. See if you can connect with optimal breathing and relax the weight of the body toward the floor; feel the earth beneath you and the contact between the body and the surface on which you're resting, and reassure yourself that you're safe in the room. Remind yourself these feelings will soon pass. In the long term, learning awareness skills, especially breathing skills, can help you to feel in control of panic and anxiety.

Feeling More Tired and Achy after the Practice

Sometimes when people first learn the body scan they feel more tired and achy afterward. When I first started practicing it, I often felt as if I'd been run over by a train by the end! It was hard to understand because all I had done was lie down and remain still, but gradually I realized that I felt worse because I was getting in touch with accumulated tension. I had been a master of blocking off from the pain, so when the walls of resistance and holding came down, for a time I was flooded by unpleasant sensations. If this is your experience, the important thing is not to give up. Keep doing the practice regularly and consistently;

over time the store of tension will gradually dissolve, and the practice becomes more pleasurable. This has certainly been my experience, and these days I generally find the body scan to be very enjoyable.

This emphasis on long-term commitment applies to any meditative practice. The way change happens is subtle, even mysterious, and it's important to avoid getting caught up with expectations of a particular outcome or short-term gain from the practice. The main thing is just to do the body scan. If you feel a little worse after doing it, never mind, and if you feel better at the end, never mind. Just keep doing it with a long-term perspective, and over time you'll realize the benefits in every aspect of life. The body scan provides a period of rest and renewal that helps you to have more energy and vitality, no matter how you felt within the period of practice itself.

CHAPTER 14

Mindfulness of Breathing

Body like a mountain;
Heart like the ocean;
Mind like the sky.
ZEN MEDITATION INSTRUCTION

The mindfulness of breathing meditation practice is the next step in using mindfulness to manage pain and illness. It builds on the skills developed in the body scan and applies them in a more precise and detailed way. The mindfulness of breathing meditation teaches you how to:

- Use the breath to inhabit the body with awareness and soften tension and resistance.
- Pay attention to one thing at a time by using each breath as an object of focus or awareness. This is naturally calming.
- Cultivate a broad and deep perspective in which you notice how your breath, physical sensations, thoughts, and emotions all come into being and pass away, moment by moment. This helps to deepen an inner sense of stability and balance as you relate to them in a more fluid and pliant way.

CONNECTING TO THE BODY AND THE MOMENT

In the mindfulness of breathing, the main object of attention is the natural breath as it flows into and out of the body. As I've said, this is a fantastic way to be in touch with the body while anchored in the present moment.

THE PRACTICE

Posture

While doing the body scan you may have begun to associate meditation with lying down, and sometimes people feel reluctant to start sitting up to meditate. I used to think it didn't matter and that if someone's health condition meant that it was more comfortable to meditate when lying down, they should do so. But it's much easier to be alert and awake when sitting than when lying down, so now that we're moving on to the mindfulness of breathing I suggest that you should at least have a go at sitting for meditation. If you find it too uncomfortable, then of course it's fine to continue to meditate lying down. But you never know—you might find it's not as difficult as you think, and the benefits of increased alertness may outweigh any increase in pain you feel.

The following short exercise will give you a sense of the power of breath awareness (an audio version is also available on the Sounds True website: soundstrue.com/burch).

EXERCISE: MINDFULNESS OF BREATHING

Adopt a comfortable posture, sitting upright if you can, and let your body settle onto the surface on which you are resting. Tune in to a broad sense of how you're feeling with an attitude of kind curiosity.

Gradually gather your awareness around the movements of your breath and body. Pay particular attention to the swelling and subsiding of the belly. Notice how the movements are continually changing, and rest your awareness within this flow of sensations.

Keeping this breath awareness as an anchor, notice the thoughts that are going through your mind and any emotions. Allow these thoughts and emotions to rise and fall like waves on the ocean, and notice they're continually changing, just like the breath.

Stay here for a few moments, and each time your mind wanders, gently bring it back to the breath and the body.

The Method

There are various ways to do the mindfulness of breathing, including the unstructured approach of the exercise above, but I find it helpful to follow a traditional method that has four stages of roughly equal length. For example, if you're meditating for twenty minutes, you can do four stages of about five minutes each. In each stage you rest your awareness on the sensations of the natural breath as it moves in and out of the body. Don't try to alter the breath in any way; simply let the breath come and go in a natural rhythm and rest your awareness on the body's sensations as it responds to the flow of the breath. Remember, breathing isn't an idea; it's a physical experience that takes place throughout the body. (For a led version of this four-stage practice see page 270.)

Stage One

The mind often settles more easily at the start of a period of meditation if it has something to do, so as an aid to staying engaged it can be helpful to count the breaths, saying each number silently. In the first stage, count at the end of each breath, from one to ten, until you've counted ten breaths; then start again at one, as follows:

- Breathe in, breathe out, and say "one."
- Breathe in, breathe out, and say "two."
- Continue in this way until you breathe in, breathe out, and say "ten."
- Then start again at "one."

A traditional image for this stage of the practice is to imagine you're a cow herder counting cattle as they pass through a gate from one field into another. As the first cow passes through, you count "one" after it has passed into the new field; you then continue to count each cow after it has passed through the gate.

Stage Two

The second stage is similar to the first, but you'll probably find that it requires just a little more concentration as you now anticipate each breath by counting just before each in-breath as follows:

- Say "one," breathe in, breathe out.
- Say "two," breathe in, breathe out.
- Continue in this way until you say "ten," and breathe in and breathe out.
- Then start again at "one."

A traditional image for this stage is to imagine you're counting out cups of rice from a large sack before putting them into a saucepan. You count "one" as you scoop the rice into the cup before pouring it into the pan.

At some point you'll almost certainly lose track of the counting in both these stages as the mind wanders. Each time you notice this, gently bring the mind back and start counting again from "one." You might never get beyond counting one or two breaths, or you may notice you're counting "forty-five, forty-six . . . ," and so on. Never mind. No matter how or why you've lost track, just note that it has happened and gently go back to "one" again.

AN IMAGE FOR STAGES ONE AND TWO

Imagine each number is like a pebble gently cast into a still pool of water. Between the end of each out-breath and the start of the next in-breath is a natural pause, and very lightly and gently you drop the number into the still pool of this pause. This image helps the counting to feel light and natural rather than dominating the awareness of the breath.

Stage Three

In the third stage, let go of the counting and follow the whole breathing process. As you do this, you broaden out your field of awareness and engage with all the sensations of breathing throughout the body. These sensations range from the very first contact of the air with the skin at the start of each in-breath through the gentle swelling of the chest, lungs, and belly as the breath reaches its natural fullness. Then you notice the changing sensations as the breath turns, becoming the out-breath, and when that ends, you may notice the tiny pause between breaths and rest there. The body then naturally responds as the next in-breath starts to form.

When you develop a stable and subtle awareness of the rhythm of your breathing, the experience can become quite exquisite. Awareness of the breath provides an anchor for the mind and emotions, and they tend to settle and become calm. This stage can feel restful because it encourages a sense of receptivity and openness to whatever you experience.

AN IMAGE FOR STAGE THREE

Imagine a wave flowing up and down a broad, textured sandy beach. The wave begins in the ocean and then flows up the beach until it naturally reaches its peak and comes to a moment of perfect stillness. It then turns and flows back down the beach to rejoin the ocean. The ocean then swells, hovers, and the next wave sighs into life.

Stage Four

In the fourth stage, gently refine your field of awareness to focus on a single sensation. Traditionally it's suggested that you rest your awareness on the very first and very last sensations that arise as the air enters and leaves the body, which are around the tip of the nose, or perhaps on the upper lip or just inside the nostrils. This stage comes last because the mind needs to have already cultivated a certain amount of calmness and alertness to settle on these delicate sensations.

The quality of awareness in this stage needs to be soft, yet focused, rather than fixed so tightly you feel you're going cross-eyed! The attention is alert yet light and delicate, like a bee gathering pollen with an almost weightless responsiveness to the flower, or like a spiderweb gently blowing in the breeze, or like catching a falling feather. If you try to grasp the feather, it will blow away, so instead you just open your palm and let it settle.

> ### AN IMAGE FOR STAGE FOUR
>
> Imagine a wave laps gently against a rock. Notice what happens when the wave meets the rock. The delicate sensations of the contact between the breath and the skin are like the contact between the wave and the rock: precise, delicate, continually changing. That's an image for the contact between the breath and your body.

Other Points of Focus in Stage Four

The main point of this stage is to narrow the range of sensations you're noticing, and an alternative to focusing on the tip of the nose is to rest your awareness on the rise and fall of the abdomen or the movement of the chest. Often those of us living with pain have a strongly ingrained habit of "living in our heads," and resting awareness on the nose area may reinforce this. Resting awareness on the rise and fall of the abdomen, however, can help you to feel more embodied. I suggest you experiment to see what works for you; it may be different at different times. If you are inclined toward dullness and sleepiness, it can help to place the awareness higher in the body, maybe on the nose area, as this tends to raise and brighten your energy. However, if you're restless and unsettled, placing awareness lower in the body is effective because it's naturally grounding and calming.

THE STRUCTURE OF THE PRACTICE

The four stages of the mindfulness of breathing give it a fairly formal structure. You can also do a longer version of the more open, unstructured breathing exercise described at the beginning of this chapter (see page 180). Some people like this and find it an effective way to become mindful of the breath. However, most people find the stages helpful when they're learning to meditate because they provide both form and variety.

The four stages are progressively a little more demanding. Counting after each breath in the first stage gives the mind an activity to engage with, and that helps in settling down. I find that if I just sit down and watch the breath without counting, I tend to be pulled around by thoughts and feelings related to my previous activity. I am also inclined to be more caught up with my pain and associated mental reactions. If I count, I can engage with the practice more quickly.

Counting in anticipation of each breath in the second stage requires a little more attention, so it takes you just a little deeper. You'll probably find that in this stage you need a bit more sensitivity to maintain a feeling of interest and engagement.

Some people find the counting in these stages more of a hindrance than anything else, and if that's your experience, I suggest you simply don't count. Remember, this practice is the mindfulness of breathing, not the mindfulness of counting! The counting is simply an aid that may help you settle and become more stable and still.

In the third stage you let go of counting because it's likely that by then you'll have dropped into a calmer, more stable state of body and mind. Just rest your awareness on your physical sensations, thoughts, and feelings as they rise and pass away, and maintain a sense of balance and calm. One writer describes this attitude as a "nonreactive watchful receptivity that neither suppresses the contents of experience nor compulsively reacts to them."[1] In other words, you're aware of what's happening and have an attitude of equanimity.

In the fourth stage you refine your awareness to become more focused, still, and concentrated, which is yet another important aspect of the practice.

Changing emphasis as you move from stage to stage helps you to stay interested and engaged in the practice. The transition between stages is a reminder of what you're doing and an opportunity to get back to the present moment, the body, and the breath. Offering the mind some variety helps guard against boredom and distraction while also supporting the gradual deepening of your awareness. Overall, the practice is a way of gathering up the strands of your awareness into an integrated and satisfying sense of wholeness and calm.

MICHAEL

Suffering from fibromyalgia and depression, it has been so helpful to learn to come back to the breath when I get lost in my mind. My practice often involves noticing that my mind has wandered and making the choice to come back, over and over again. Previously I felt that thoughts and emotions were dragging me away, and there was nothing I could do about it. They were so strong and emotionally laden, and they seemed very real, but meditation began to show me, *Ah, I can exercise choice and let go of my anxious thoughts*. The mindfulness of breathing has been a powerful way to put this into practice. And when I really engage with the breath and just let go, there's an extraordinary richness to the physical sensations of breath.

EXPLORING THE PRACTICE

Distraction

Even with its four stages, the technique of the mindfulness of breathing is really very simple: the stages are just different ways of resting the mind on the breath. But most people find that remaining undistractedly aware of the breath isn't as straightforward as it sounds. A common experience is that the mind and emotions quickly become interested in other things. Some of the thoughts that enter your mind will be strong and compelling; others may be vague and indistinct. Some will be pleasant and enticing, and some can even be disturbing and unsettling. Before you know it, you'll be thinking about dinner, shopping, sex, the argument you had last night, your itchy foot, your tense shoulders, the fact that you're irritated with your boss (complete with rehearsing all the things you'd like to say to him or her), and so on. At some point you'll remember, *Oh, I'm supposed to be becoming aware of the breath!* You'll bring your awareness back, and for a moment you'll be collected. But before you know it, the mind will, in all likelihood, start to wander again.

Chapter 16 contains much more discussion of how to work with various obstacles to meditation, but here I want to offer some comments to guard against any tendency to feel discouraged.

It's natural for thoughts to pop up in your mind and for you to become interested in them. Meditation won't stop this right away, so I encourage you to see it as a chance to explore your mind, heart, tendencies, habits, and propensities, and to get to know yourself more deeply rather than assume you must be doing it wrong if you're dominated by thoughts.

Each time you bring yourself back to the breath is a moment of training. This is how the heart and mind learn to move from a state of habitual and reactive distraction to one that's more responsive, creative, and aware. I can't emphasize this point enough, as it can save you from falling into feelings of failure and despondency.

DELICATE MIND

Imagine a butterfly resting on the head of a flower as it gently moves in a light breeze on a summer day. The butterfly is poised, alert, and receptive to the weight and movement of the flower, but it is also very still and quiet. You can feel your mind and heart becoming like that butterfly in meditation: each time it flutters away, it comes back to rest.

Concentration

Learning to concentrate on the sensations of breathing is good training in how to apply attention and effort. Many of us think of concentration as a chore or a burden—after all, it's what you have to do for exams or tasks you find difficult. In these instances it's often tinged with anxiety and fear. But the quality of the concentration you're learning in the mindfulness of breathing practice is warm and delicate. It's direct, yet light; focused, yet gentle.

Slowing Down

Mindfulness slows things down. Usually experience is filled with noise, conversation, activity, decisions, and so on. Then there are the layers of evaluations, views, opinions, reactions, and habits added on to experience without consciously choosing them. Living like this, we often don't know what our experience really is.

Through practicing the mindfulness of breathing, you will gradually become clearer about what's actually happening and more familiar with your habitual reactions and impulses. You can watch calmly as your physical, mental, and emotional experiences arise and pass away. Focusing on the breath anchors your awareness in the body and the present moment.

VAST MIND

Imagine you're sitting on a hilltop overlooking a vast and beautiful plain filled with birds and animals. You watch with interest what's happening on the plain without being strongly drawn to one animal or another. You may see animals such as lions or tigers that would usually scare you, but because you see them from the hilltop there's no need to run away. If you see beautiful gazelle or antelope, you enjoy their elegance and watch them with relaxed interest while remaining quiet and still.

In the mindfulness of breathing, your thoughts and feelings are like these different animals, and your field of awareness resembles the vast plain. Your pain and thoughts about the pain might be frightening, like the lions and tigers, but mindfulness offers a vantage point from which you can be aware of the pain without reacting or being driven by anxiety and fear into feeling that you have to escape.

CHAPTER 15

Kindly Awareness

Just as a mother protects with her life
Her child, her only child,
So, with boundless hearts
May we cherish all living beings,
Radiating kindness throughout the world.

THE BUDDHA[1]

With the body scan and mindfulness of breathing as a basis, we can move on to the third meditation practice, which is the heart of the approach to mindfulness that we've developed at Breathworks. The kindly awareness practice, adapted from a traditional Buddhist meditation practice called "the development of loving-kindness" (*mettabhavana*), is concerned with kindness and empathy, which in turn bring peace and stability of heart and mind.

THE PRACTICE

In the practice there are five stages in which you bring kindly awareness to yourself, a friend, someone you don't know well, someone you find difficult, and all living things. Each stage is underpinned by several other elements: a kindly attitude and intention, kindly breath, seeing the shared patterns of our lives, and a balanced attitude toward pleasure and pain. I'll explore these elements further at the end of the chapter.

Stage One: Responding Kindly to the Whole of Your Experience

Although the practice is about empathizing with others, the first stage is spent cultivating kindness toward yourself and awareness of your own experience. This might seem surprising, even selfish, but it's only really possible to connect with others if you are first able to connect with yourself with awareness, openness, and honesty.

Kindly Breath

We start by settling in to a broad experience of the body, the breath, and the moment. Bringing a sense of warmth and kindliness to the breath, imagine it soothes the body as it flows in and out. If you can't connect with a sense of kindness, simply breathe with the intention of responding kindly.

Opening to the Unpleasant

Once you're settled, gently turn your awareness toward the unpleasant side of your current experience; it's an unavoidable part of life. If you have strong sensations of pain, gently open your awareness to them with sensitivity and kindness. Should the pain or disquiet be predominantly mental or emotional, look for its echo in the body — for example, if you're anxious, this might be echoed as tension in the stomach. Bringing awareness to these physical echoes of your feelings helps you stay grounded in the present moment. (There's more on this in chapter 16: Managing Thoughts and Emotions, see page 201.)

It may seem odd, even masochistic, to take your attention to painful or unpleasant aspects of your experience at the start of the practice, but we do this for good reasons. When most of us sit down to meditate, the first thing we do, often unconsciously, is harden ourselves against anything that's unpleasant in an effort to try and block it out. We think, *Okay, I'm going to meditate. I've got a bit of pain, but I'm not going to feel that because I don't want to acknowledge it. I don't like it, and I want to have a good meditation.* In trying to exclude pain from your awareness, you set up a resistance that rapidly brings secondary suffering. This manifests as physical tension, dullness of the mind, unwillingness to sit still, irritation, and so on.

Rather than thinking, *Oh no, not that backache again — it's not fair; I can't stand it!* gently acknowledge the pain. *Okay, I'm experiencing backache — it's really painful. Breathe in; breathe out. The pain is difficult, but it's part of my experience. Let's see what it feels like.*

You can soften resistance to the unpleasant side of your experience by taking the breath to the painful sensations, breathing in softness and breathing out with a sense that you're letting go of resistance. Treat your pain as you would treat a child or someone you really love who is injured.

Another reason for starting the practice by opening to pain or discomfort is to make sure you keep the heart soft and open. If your initial reflex is to harden yourself against pain, you'll find that you are, in fact, hardening your awareness to a whole band of sensitivity that includes pleasure, love, and the potential you have to be fully and vibrantly alive.

Seeking the Pleasant

After you have sat with unpleasant, difficult, or painful sensations or experiences for a time, focus now on the pleasurable aspects of the moment. For example, you might become more aware of the warmth of your hands, or something as simple as the fact that you're not hungry. You may notice relief around your heart as you relax into an honest acceptance of the moment instead of the hardness that goes with resisting it.

Some people find it difficult to experience subtle sensations, in which case look for feelings of energy in the body or enjoy the simple process of breathing. You aren't necessarily looking for a big or grand experience; simply rest your awareness on anything pleasurable in your experience with an attitude of kindly curiosity.

Becoming a Bigger Container

Having explored the painful and pleasant sides of your experience, broaden your perspective on it to become a "bigger container" that's able to hold the pleasant and painful aspects of the moment with equanimity. When you notice you're tipping into aversion or craving, drop back to your emotional center again and continue to sit with the flow of experience. Within this broad, integrated awareness you can now investigate the nature of experience. Living *with* life's continual changes instead of fighting against them creates strength and stability. And all the time the practice is held by the kindly breath, soothing and caressing all of your experience.

It may feel challenging to look directly at unpleasant experiences or it may feel impossible to find anything pleasant. For more on the issues raised by this stage of the practice, look again at the discussion of the five-step process in chapter 5.

✵ JEMMA

When I first practiced the kindly awareness meditation, I completely missed the point of the first stage. I filtered out the importance of being kind toward myself as a basis for being kind to others. I suppose it's because I didn't want to accept my back pain, and I didn't want to admit I needed help, so I tended to think that everybody else was worse off than me. It has been a deep relief to change from pushing myself to being kind to myself and more aware of how I feel. I have feelings and emotions, just as other people do. That has given me a sense of connectedness with other people.

Stage Two: A Good Friend

In the second stage of the practice, bring to mind a friend. While you're learning the practice it's best to choose someone to whom you aren't sexually attracted, who is roughly your own age, and who is alive. This is to avoid introducing more complicated feelings that come with sexual desire, parent-child dynamics, or grief.

Invite this person into your awareness in whatever way feels most alive and engaged. This may be through a mental image or a feeling of what he or she is like. A memory can sometimes help evoke the friend, but take care not to get carried away by it: *It was lovely being on the beach with Katie. We had ice cream and met that nice guy. What was his name again?* Before you know it, you're lost in associative stories. When you notice your attention has wandered, just come back to the kindly breath and a simple sense of your friend.

Once you've evoked a sense of your friend, sit with your experience of this person and bring to mind what you share. In the first stage you reflected on the pleasure and pain in your own experience; now reflect that in each moment of your friend's life, he or she also feels pain and resists the experience, and feels pleasure and tries to cling to it. The stories of our lives are different, but the basic human experience is similar. Just like you, your friend feels joy and sorrow, hope and fear, and experiences triumphs and regrets. Your friend experiences the same range of emotions that you have, and like you, he or she wants to love and be loved.

You can also reflect that, just like you, your friend is breathing in and out, and that each breath is unique and brings life to his or her body just as your breath is at the heart of your life. Introduce kindness to the breath: on the in-breath being aware of your friend and his or her humanity, and on the out-breath breathing out kindness and an intention of well-wishing toward your friend. Everything you wish for yourself you can wish for your friend.

Stage Three: A Neutral Person

In the third stage, bring to mind someone for whom you have no feelings of like or dislike, perhaps because you don't know this person well. The neutral person represents the vast mass of humanity about whom you usually don't think very much. You may even relate to him or her as an object rather than a fellow human being. Choose someone you know by sight, such as a local shopkeeper or someone in your life with whom you haven't formed an emotional connection, someone who works at the office, perhaps.

Bring this person to mind in a similar way as in the previous stage, and then reflect on your shared humanity with its pleasures and pains, hopes and fears. You can also reflect that, like you, this person is breathing. Introduce a quality of kindness and interest to the breath. On the in-breath become aware of this person and his or her humanity; on the out-breath breathe out kindness and well-wishing toward him or her.

Stage Four: A Person with Whom You Have Difficulty

In the fourth stage, bring to mind someone with whom you feel some kind of difficulty or disharmony. When you're learning the practice, it's probably best to choose someone with whom the difficulty is fairly mild or with whom you experience some irritation rather than an archenemy. Otherwise you might find yourself overwhelmed by feelings of anger or dislike and struggle to stay engaged with the meditation.

Using your imagination, connect with this person's humanity. That means reaching over your sense of separation and focusing on what you share. Reflect that, whatever difficulties there may be between you, this person also experiences the same range of emotions and longs to love and be loved. Although he or she might be difficult for you to be with, in fact you share the same tendencies of avoiding the unpleasant and grasping the pleasant, along with the behavior that springs from this. You aren't so different after all.

Instead of your response being dominated by dislike, you may start to see this person in a new light, with a broader, kinder, more empathetic perspective. In this stage, too, you can infuse the breath with kindness. On the in-breath you become aware of this person; on the out-breath you breathe out kindness and well-wishing.

Stage Five: Spreading Kindness Universally

In the final stage, bring to mind the four people you've already thought of: yourself, the friend, the neutral person, and the person you find difficult. Imagine you're sitting together in a circle — or you might just have a sense of the four people and connect with an awareness of all that you share.

Now broaden your awareness further to include an ever-widening circle of people. You can reflect that every human being experiences the same mixture of pain and pleasure as you, no matter where you live, your age, color, or wealth, or any other perceived difference. Allow kindly awareness to permeate your breath as you think of a widening circle of life. You may sense the whole world breathing and rising and falling, like waves on the ocean. As the hard edges of separation soften, let go into a sense of connection with life and rest quietly with the kindly breath.

Gradually bring the practice to a close, noticing sounds and sensations in the body. When you feel ready, open your eyes, gently move your body, and reengage with the day.

CHOOSING PEOPLE FOR THE STAGES

When you choose the people to reflect on in the second, third, and fourth stages of the practice, it's good to decide quickly instead of worrying about whether you have the right person. You may find that people move around the stages, and someone who's in the "good friend" stage one day is in the "difficult person" category the next! This is normal—everybody has ups and downs in their relationships. It's also fine if the same person stays in a stage for days, weeks, or even months, and this can be a good way to build up your practice.

It's important to remember that you are not trying to change the other person in this practice. Although you'll find that your relationships alter over time, this will be because you're relating to people differently, perhaps becoming kinder and less judgmental as a result of practicing the kindly awareness meditation. You can never make another person change; you can only take responsibility for your own responses and behavior.

ELEMENTS OF THE PRACTICE

Several key attitudes run through all the stages of the kindly awareness practice and I'd like to explore these in greater depth.

An Attitude of Kindness and Connection

A word that beautifully evokes the attitude to your experience that we encourage in the kindly awareness practice is *tender*. The dictionary defines *tender* as "easily damaged, vulnerable or sensitive; kind, merciful or sympathetic; touching; having or expressing warm and affectionate feelings; gentle and delicate; requiring care in handling."[2] It suggests loving and caring, plus also knowing the right amount of care to offer someone.

As you practice, you will gradually learn to distinguish what might be called "perfunctory awareness" — which is cool and detached — and "emotionally engaged awareness," something you cultivate in this practice. It's warm, honest, and kind.

Intention

What happens if you do the practice when you aren't feeling kind? Trying to conjure up an emotion is bound to feel artificial, but the practice is really about how you approach and engage with yourself and others. The key is that you have an *intention* to make a positive connection with others, and simply breathing in and out with such an intention of kindness can be surprisingly powerful.

When a gardener plants seeds in the earth, at first there's nothing to show for them. But in time the seeds will sprout and bloom. The intention to respond kindly to others also bears fruit in due course, whatever you may feel while you're doing the practice.

Kindly Breath

Breath awareness is the foundation of the kindly awareness practice, as it is of the body scan and the mindfulness of breathing. In this practice you connect breath awareness with an emotional attitude that's warm and kindly, especially when you become aware of pain. Encourage a tender, gentle awareness to permeate the breath, so the breath itself helps you soften any resistance. In the first stage of the practice this means *breathing in with awareness* of your experience and then *breathing out kindness toward your experience,* allowing it to permeate the body. In the second stage you breathe in awareness of your friend, and on the out-breath, breathe out kindness toward them, and so on in the other stages.

A Balanced Attitude Toward Pleasure and Pain

Learning to be aware of the unpleasant and pleasant dimensions of your experience is a key to uncoupling your immediate experience from your reactions to it. This allows space for a more creative response, and instead of being buffeted by your responses to pain and pleasure you'll experience greater equanimity and stability. Just as sailors place ballast—heavy material such as sand or rocks—in the keel of a boat to prevent it from capsizing, your emotional ballast enables you to correct your balance by resting in a broad and stable field of awareness. You feel like a streamlined yacht that carves a clean course through the sea rather than a tiny dinghy bobbing about at the mercy of each wave. It also helps in stabilizing your experience to feel that your emotional and physical energy is based low in the body instead of identifying with the thoughts and emotions rushing around your head.

Regularly practicing the kindly awareness meditation helps to embed this way of relating to experience in your daily habits. Gradually you learn to catch the "tipping point" when a simple unpleasant experience hardens into resistance and avoidance, or a pleasant feeling is crushed by your urgent desire to hold on to it. As Jon Kabat-Zinn says, "You don't have to freak out when your buttons are pushed."[3] There are many opportunities to get irritated—life is like that! But if you are mindful and aware, and see more deeply into your moment-by-moment experience, you can notice the freaking out impulse, the tipping point, and recontact your ballast and stability.

Diaries of Pleasant and Unpleasant Events

Many people find that it helps to keep diaries of pleasant and unpleasant events during the week prior to starting the kindly awareness practice. Templates for these diaries are in appendix 2. Each day, you note an event that you found pleasant or unpleasant and the physical, mental, and emotional responses it prompted. You'll probably notice how varied and textured your day-to-day experience really is, even if you tend to think that it's dominated by pain. The diaries also reveal that your life includes simple pleasures to which you may normally pay little attention, and you can see at a glance how quickly secondary suffering can follow pain or difficulty.

Seeing the Shared Patterns of Our Lives

As well as helping you to notice your own tendencies to resist pain and cling to pleasure, through kindly awareness you also notice them in other people. In fact, this is the human condition. In the kindly awareness practice you reflect on the way your reactions cause you to suffer, and this enables you to empathize with the pain others feel whenever they are pierced by the arrows of secondary suffering. Rather than reacting to other people's behavior, such reflections help you understand them, and this brings empathy and tolerance. You move from isolation, when you're focused on how different you are from others — an especially strong tendency for those of us living with pain — to connectedness, when you're aware of the shared patterns of our lives. The details of our lives are unique, but the basic human experience is very similar.

CHAPTER 16

Managing Thoughts and Emotions

Now that you have been introduced to the basic principles of meditation and the structure of the practices, it's time to look at how to work with your experience in each meditation session, particularly how to manage thoughts and emotions.

MANAGING THOUGHTS

It is commonly thought that meditation means to not think, or even to empty the mind. Let's clear this up right away. It's perfectly normal to think — that's what the mind does. So, with the exception of very refined meditation states, thoughts will always be present in your meditation. The question isn't "How do I get rid of thoughts?" but "How do I work effectively with thoughts and change my relationship with them?" In mindfulness meditation you don't try to push thoughts away or wall yourself off from them. Instead, the aim is to be aware of whatever is happening moment by moment, including your thoughts, with a nonreactive attitude.

When you meditate you may find that various thought processes occupy your mind, dominating it with almost shocking intensity. It can even seem as if you're thinking more than you were before. That's unlikely; you're just becoming more aware of what was there already, beneath the radar of your awareness. The constant rumble of thoughts is like the background noise of a washing machine, which often you won't notice until it starts the spin cycle. Whenever you meditate, the thoughts you notice will have been rumbling away beyond your awareness, influencing your actions and emotions. You may feel tension in your body prompted by anxious thoughts that you haven't fully registered, or you could feel depressed without knowing why or how to change it — but you haven't noticed that going a round your mind are angry thoughts about your pain and illness. These are examples of being on autopilot, and it's how most of us live, most of the time. Only when you become aware of these thoughts can you take responsibility for how you respond to them, and one of the main purposes of meditation is to be mindful of thoughts and to find creative ways of relating to them.

Looking at Thoughts, Rather Than from Them

Usually, when you have a thought, you tend to believe what it's telling you and to look at the world *from* the point of view of the thought. But mindfulness of thoughts means looking *at* your thoughts rather than *from* them. For example, imagine you're doing the body scan and you think, *I can't do this, I may as well give up.* It's easy to believe what that thought is telling you, but if you notice it's just a thought, not objective truth, it loses its power. You can let the thought be and carry on with the body scan. It's important to remember that thoughts are not facts — even those that say they are![1] This doesn't mean everything you think is untrue; it's just that not everything you think is true, *and* some things are untrue *and* unhelpful. Mindfulness helps you to notice your thoughts without taking them at face value or buying in to them.[2]

❋ **TOM**

I get migraines that are followed by two days of feeling absolutely drained. One of the best ways of dealing with them is to bring mindfulness to my thoughts. I would have overwhelming thoughts such as, *Not something else to deal with! Will my physical problems never end?* But if I just let these thoughts come and go, and remember they are *not* facts, just thoughts that I *think* are true, my thinking is transformed. I see they aren't helpful, so I don't buy into them. If I treat the migraines with kindness, knowing that, as with all things, they will come and go, a wonderful sense of peace arises.

Emotionally Charged Thoughts

Your ability to notice thoughts without believing in them depends in part on the nature of the thought. Some thoughts are fairly trivial and don't have a strong emotional charge.[3] If you're meditating and the thought occurs, *What shall I have for lunch today?* it's easy to notice that and let it go. Other thoughts are more urgent, though still fairly trivial. *I mustn't forget to send a birthday card to Bill* readily prompts the thought, *I must write Bill's birthday card now.* It can be hard to resist the urge to get up and write the card there and then, although the truth is that you could write it later. If you notice the thought *as a thought,* you can decide how to respond rather than finding yourself writing the card without having decided consciously to stop meditating! If you're often bothered by "I must remember" thoughts, keep a pen and paper beside you as you meditate and write them down. You can then let the thought go and get back to meditating.

Some thoughts have a strong emotional charge, and it's harder to notice these thoughts as thoughts. The thought, *What if the lump on my neck is cancer?* is likely to prompt worry and anxiety, and it's hard to just sit with that. But you can still notice the thought and the associated emotions and also be aware of how you turn them into a drama. *I bet it's cancer — my aunt had a lump in her neck that was cancer. I won't be able to cope. Who will look after the children if I die?* In this example, a simple observation — a lump that may be harmless — has ended up in speculation that *I'm going to die.*

Catastrophizing

Another word for this tendency is *catastrophizing,* and it's a common tendency for those of us living with pain and illness. It's easy to over-identify with one element in your experience and lose all perspective.

One of my meditation teachers told me that when he was a little boy, if he fell over and got the knees of his trousers dirty, he would wail to his mother, "I'm dirty!" He called this the "I'm-dirty-all-over syndrome" because that's how he saw himself even though there was only a small patch of mud on his knees. You easily overidentify with the part of your experience that's painful as if it were everything, when it may only be that a small part of your back hurts, for example.

We can also catastrophize about new pains. Recently in a Breathworks course, Sylvia talked about a stomach pain that had developed. She worried about it incessantly, and she told us that, "By the end of the day I was dead and buried and attending my own funeral!" She'd been taken over by a catastrophizing thought process, engaging with it as if it were fact, and spent hours absorbed in a self-destructive fantasy.

Thoughts like these are compelling, and if you try to suppress them you'll probably become tense and tired. Mindfulness means learning to notice these thoughts for what they are—just thoughts, not reality—and coming back to your immediate felt experience of the present moment and the body, remembering that each moment is multifaceted and contains more than just your pain. This enables you to interrupt the stories you tell yourself and develop greater emotional robustness.

The Problem with Buying In to Thoughts

Often buying in to a thought is relatively harmless. For example, it won't do too much damage if you stop meditating and write Bill's birthday card, but other thoughts can cause you to suffer unnecessarily if you believe them. For instance, you might have the thought, *I've got so much to do at work, I'll never get it all done.* This may be untrue but if you believe it, you can feel stressed. Or you may be trying to do something difficult and have the thought, *This is too hard—I can't do it.* This could even apply to meditating: *I can't meditate—I'm no good at it.* Again, this may not be true, but if you believe it, you might give up, which can give rise to another thought: *I'm no good at anything.* That's definitely untrue, but it can prompt yet another thought that says, *I'm worthless*. Before you know it, you're feeling depressed.

It's especially important for those of us dealing with pain and illness to see thoughts for what they are, as we already have a lot to deal with. If your thoughts are spiraling out of control, you may quickly find yourself feeling miserable. The good news is that you can maintain perspective and balance by becoming aware. The box that follows offers some helpful ways to view your thoughts.

IMAGES FOR LOOKING AT THOUGHTS RATHER THAN FROM THEM

THE THOUGHT TRAIN

Imagine you're standing on a bridge, looking down at a freight train with open cars that are slowly moving along the track. Each of the cars is a thought, and your job is to watch them go past—now you're looking at your thoughts. But from time to time you lose your awareness and jump off the bridge into one of the cars and get carried away down the line by that thought—now you're looking from a thought.[4]

A THEATER

You're sitting in the audience of a theater. Actors enter from the right of the stage, one at a time, walking across it and exiting stage left. Imagine these actors are thoughts and you're letting them pass across the stage.[5]

SKY AND CLOUDS

The sky is your mind, and the clouds are the thoughts that come and go. Some may be small, white clouds while others could be big, black ones. Some may be so big that at times they cover the whole sky. But you never forget that the blue sky behind the clouds is always there, even if you can't see it.

LEAVES ON A STREAM

You're sitting on a rock in the middle of a stream looking at the water. It's autumn, and the leaves are falling from overhanging branches onto the water. Imagine the leaves are your thoughts. You watch the leaves as they pass by, letting them be, without interfering with their journey down the stream.

Labeling Thoughts

Another way to get some distance from thoughts is to label them. Note the type of thought they express—for example, "planning," "worrying," "rehearsing," "judging," "fantasizing," "criticizing," "remembering," and so on. This is a powerful way to defuse the emotional charge of the thought and to maintain perspective by looking *at* the thought rather than *from* the thought.

Let's say you're doing the mindfulness of breathing and notice that you're thinking: *I bet I fail my driving test tomorrow. I can't remember the rule to apply when turning into traffic. What about hill starts? Oh God, I can't remember anything; it's going to be a disaster!* You notice the thought process and label it "worrying, catastrophizing." Then you can return to the body, the breath, and the present moment.

Or imagine you're doing the body scan and the feeling of relaxation triggers a thought process: *I must book an osteopathy session. It was so amazing when I had the last treatment. Peter really loosened up my neck. It was such a nice room, too—calm and quiet. Wouldn't it be nice to have coffee in the bar down the road?* The practice is to catch yourself and to drop in the labels "remembering" and "fantasizing." Then you can go back to the body scan.

When I started using this method, I identified a habit of rehearsing events in advance. I realized that ever since I was a child I'd spent hours planning what I would say in advance of situations, especially ones that made me anxious, although even when the moment arrived I rarely said anything I'd rehearsed. I realized I could halt the process by labeling it "rehearsing."

It's important to note these thought categories lightly and without judgment while remaining emotionally engaged with your experience. The mind is just doing what minds do, and you can even develop a sense of humor about it. I often find my mind amusing!

Locating Thoughts in the Body

Another helpful method to avoid getting carried away by mind-created stories is to identify where a thought is located in the body. You may think that thoughts are stored in the head, but if you pay close attention you'll probably notice a relationship between thoughts and physical sensations. If you have the anxious thought, *I have to get this job finished to meet my deadline,* and pay attention to what's happening physically, you'll probably notice some tension associated with it—maybe a tightness in the stomach, shallow breath, or a clenched jaw.

The way thoughts are expressed physically varies between individuals, but there's always a strong relationship between the mind and the body. Sometimes you may feel as if you can't get any perspective on a thought process. But if you can locate its expression in the body and bring your awareness to those sensations, you're likely to feel grounded in the body and the moment and automatically feel some distance from the thought. If you relax the affected part of the body, you may find that the thoughts also relax a little. This feedback system undermines the power of the thought: as you relax the body, the mind relaxes, and this in turn relaxes the body.

What About Creative Thoughts?

Sometimes as the mind quiets in meditation, helpful and creative insights can come into your mind. As the mind clears, you may see the answer to a problem that's been worrying you or sense a shaft of insight into major life questions. Sometimes I've had thoughts that gave me perspective on my disability or on how my situation affects my friends and family, and these have led to feelings of empathy and love.

Thoughts like these are very positive, but within meditation the practice is to let even these thoughts come and go without getting caught up in them. Each of the meditation practices in this book has a clear focus, such as the body, the breath, or the person to whom you're directing kindly awareness. Whatever thoughts arise, the benefits of the practice will come if you continue to follow the structure of the meditation. You can think about your life another time, but you can't easily do a body scan or the mindfulness of breathing except when you're meditating! Every time you become aware of a thought, just note it mentally and come back to the breath, the body, and the moment. I recommend setting time aside each day outside of meditation to quietly reflect on your life and come back to any creative thoughts you noticed while meditating. You might also keep a journal or talk things through with a friend, and in that way the fruits of meditation can affect your whole life.

EMOTIONS—WORKING WITH STRONG EMOTIONAL STATES

Thoughts and emotions are closely related. The examples of disturbing thoughts I gave earlier in this chapter all had an emotional component. The thought, *What shall I have for lunch today?* is prompted by longing and desire. *I mustn't forget to send a birthday card to Bill* has a tinge of anxiety about it and maybe worry that Bill won't like you anymore if you forget his birthday. *What if the lump I found on my neck is cancer?* springs from outright fear.

As you become aware of thoughts as a distinct part of your experience instead of being lost in what you're thinking about (the thought's content), your emotions will slowly become more manageable. You can also work directly with emotional states, which will influence your thoughts because emotions and thoughts continually affect one another. Many emotions can affect your meditation, and you may be amazed at how many emotions it is possible to experience, even within a short space of time. This is a perfectly normal part of the process of being alive.

But mindfulness meditation isn't about getting rid of difficult emotions or artificially generating superficially positive ones; it means becoming more aware of your experience in each moment, including your emotions. Just as thoughts arise and pass, an emotion too is a transitory experience, and just as you can easily buy in to the content of thoughts, you easily experience emotions as an all-consuming reality. But if you can mindfully notice constricted emotional states, they tend to soften. This looser relationship with your emotions creates space for more relaxed, calm, and positive feelings to naturally blossom and grow. Here again is the magical, alchemical dimension of awareness.

IMAGES FOR EMOTIONAL DISTURBANCES

If the settled, calm mind is like a still lake of clear water, then disturbing emotions disrupt the water in various ways:

- Anger, hatred, and rage are like water that's boiling.
- Desire and craving are like water that's colored by seductive dyes.
- Anxiety, restlessness, and worry are like water that's whipped up into choppy waves by the wind.
- Sluggishness, depression, and despondency are like water that's clogged with weeds.
- Doubt and lack of confidence are like water that's stagnant and dirty.

I find these images helpful when meditating. Identifying the type of emotional state I'm experiencing and the way it's disturbing the clear water of the mind gives me perspective. I can look at the emotion instead of being identified with it. Then I can allow the turbulent water to settle, so it can gradually return to stillness and clarity.[6]

The Middle Way Between Overidentification and Suppression

Being mindfully aware of emotions means finding a middle way between overidentifying with their content and pushing away or suppressing them. If you find you're overidentifying with an emotion such as fear, you can broaden out your field of awareness to include the body and the breath; if you're cutting off from an emotion, leaving you blocked and dry, you can move toward it. You might do this by exploring the sensations in the body connected with the emotion (seeing where the fear is expressed physically, for example), or resting your awareness in the heart area with softness and care. It can be fascinating to work with emotional states in this way, learning when you need to back off and when to move closer.

Meditation as Familiarization

If you experience a disturbing emotion while meditating, it's easy to feel despondent. Keep going! This is what it means to get to know the heart and mind. It helps to see meditation as something that will change you in the long term rather than to judge it in a single session from your ups and downs. The Tibetan word for meditation means "familiarization."[7] This suggests meditation is about becoming more aware of what makes you tick and more familiar with the tendencies of the heart and mind. Whatever you experience is an opportunity for learning. If things are difficult and you get in a state, at least you can avoid getting into a state about *being* in a state! The bedrock of meditation is present-moment awareness of the body and the breath, and you can always come back to these grounding and reassuring presences.

Sometimes an entire session of meditation may consist of being carried away by fear, noticing this, coming back to the body, breathing a calming breath, bouncing off into fear again, noticing this, coming back to the body, and so on. This might not feel pleasant, but it would be a highly effective period of meditation. Bringing awareness to your experience is much healthier than trying to block out the fear or spiraling into rumination and anxiety. Learning to sit with strong emotions in a grounded way is tremendous training for all aspects of life.

On a retreat some years ago I was assailed by fear and confusion. Every meditation session was dominated by strong emotions and thoughts that spiraled out of control. I sweated with nervous perspi-ration, had diarrhea, lost weight, and experienced palpitations. Each night I lay in bed unable to sleep, and I felt angry and humiliated by what was happening. I started to fear the fear, an escalating spiral, and I didn't know how to manage it. A friend helped by saying that I was probably experiencing fear of the unknown because I was in an unfamiliar inner landscape. It would never be this bad again because next time I'd have more self-knowledge to guide me.

My friend was right. Fear and insecurity have sometimes come up as a primary experience, but having familiarized myself with my mental and emotional landscape through years of meditation, I am now able to sit with these feelings without panicking or falling into the complex reactions that produce secondary suffering. This gives me confidence and stability, which are among the greatest gifts of meditation. With steady practice you learn to hold your mental and emotional experiences more lightly, no matter how intense they are, and to rest back in the flow of life, enjoying your experience as it comes into being and passes away.

You can also feel positive emotions such as joy and love welling up in meditation. If you let these emotions be, without grasping at them, you'll find they naturally grow — that's one of the most beautiful aspects of meditation.

The exploration of meditation in parts 4 and 5 of this book enables you to establish and maintain your own regular meditation practice and work with the distractions that will inevitably arise. If you stick with the practice, I confidently predict that you will experience the peace and ease that are the fruits of meditation. This will help you to live more in harmony with your circumstances, whatever they may be.

PART VI

Mindfulness at All Times

CHAPTER 17

Mindfulness in Daily Life

I n this chapter I'll suggest ways to bring mindfulness into the nitty-gritty of daily activity. Meditation and mindful movement are essential foundations of mindfulness training, but the key to living well with pain and illness is being able to maintain this awareness in ordinary activities. This isn't easy, and you'll need to look closely at your deepest habits if you are to sustain mindfulness outside the structures of the formal practices I've introduced in the previous chapters.

ALIGNING YOUR ASPIRATIONS WITH YOUR REALITY

One of the most crucial challenges is aligning your aspirations — what you set out to achieve — with an accurate sense of your circumstances. It takes time to gradually orient your life in a direction that has meaning for you and is also realistic, given your health.

When I was first living with pain and disability, I habitually behaved in ways that made it worse. Because I was frustrated, I would move furniture, carry heavy shopping bags, try to climb mountains, and sit at my computer for hours at a time. Day after day I ended up feeling wrecked, and I would lie on my bed in despair, thinking, *If only I could get to the point where I no longer want to do the things that harm me.* That seemed an impossible dream as my personal aspirations and values were still tied up with being a fit and active person rather than the person living with pain that I actually was. Kerry, a young woman with a severe chronic condition, describes her own similar experience.

> ❋ **KERRY**
>
> I did well in my exams at university, and I want to get my degree and make a life for myself despite my health problems, but I can't seem to find the balance between looking after myself and achieving my goals. Looking after my back seems to involve sacrificing many of my aspirations, and my aspirations seem to conflict with my condition. I feel good when I achieve something, but then guilty when it's at the cost of increased pain. I feel more positive about myself when I listen to my body and keep my pain to a minimum, but then I feel that life's passing me by, and I'm being left behind.

I feel for Kerry and other young people I've met through my courses, but I tell them that through consistent mindfulness training it's possible to align one's dreams with life as it is. I take heart from the fact that, on the whole, the things I want to do with my life these days are beneficial rather than harmful to my body. I no longer even *want* to climb mountains! Letting go of that dream seemed impossible twenty years ago, but it has imperceptibly been replaced by love of meditation and exploring the *inner* world. Now I experience more meaning and fulfillment than ever, and I can live sustainably *with* the body I have, rather than *in spite* of it.

You may find that your values and aspirations naturally change as you practice mindfulness and become more self-aware. It's important to listen to your inner voice. You could decide to change your career or take up a hobby, or you might realize you've squeezed pleasurable activities out of your life and decide to rekindle old interests. What's important is to have the courage to follow your heart in a way that's aligned with your physical condition and to set up a realistic lifestyle to support your aspirations.

THE BOOM-AND-BUST CYCLE

The first thing to do is to look at some basic tendencies. A common tendency for those of us living with pain and illness is to overdo things when we feel good, causing our symptoms to flare up as a consequence. Before you know it, you're caught in a cycle of being overactive one day and then underactive the next, which plays havoc with your ability to lead a normal life. In pain management, this swing from one extreme to the other is called the "overactivity–underactivity cycle" or "boom and bust" (see figure 33).

The pattern for most of us is that we decrease activities when the pain is bad, possibly making us bedridden, and then when we have a good patch where we are able to do all the things we haven't been able to get on with, we end up overdoing it. You lose fitness while resting, so you're more likely to strain the body when you become active, and this leads to more pain. Over time flare-ups can increase, and fitness deteriorates; on top of this you feel fear, anxiety, and frustration. This

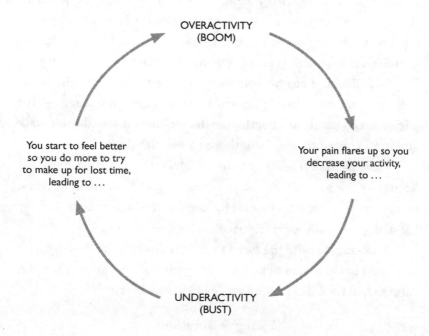

OVERACTIVITY
(BOOM)

You start to feel better
so you do more to try
to make up for lost time,
leading to . . .

Your pain flares up so you
decrease your activity,
leading to . . .

UNDERACTIVITY
(BUST)

FIGURE 33: BOOM-AND-BUST CYCLE

cycle can repeat itself many times a day, or it may play itself out over days or weeks. (This is a behavioral version of blocking and drowning, the two poles of secondary suffering that I introduced in chapter 3.)

You may also find yourself stuck in tendencies of fear and avoidance. Because you're frightened of doing anything that causes pain, you avoid such activities, perhaps avoiding virtually any activity at all. Each time you try to get back on your feet, the pain and fear are even worse, and so you decrease your activity even more. Before long, your life can be extremely limited. You hate your condition — which seems to dominate your life — and you can feel you've lost control. I know how frightening this sense of powerlessness can be.

Breaking the Cycle

In order to live well with your condition, it's vital to break out of this cycle and restore a stable and sustainable level of activity if you are to maintain your general health and well-being without overdoing things. This is called "pacing," or you may prefer to regard it as establishing a sustainable rhythm to your days. Your illness or pain problem may mean that you have to accept limitations — for example, the paralysis affecting my lower limbs means I can't walk and run as I used to, and I often need a wheelchair. But you can still find your maximum level of activity, given those limitations, and keep it as regular and varied as possible. You don't need to run a marathon; you can achieve a lot by keeping the body mobile in daily life and getting some cardiovascular exercise, such as swimming or faster walking, to raise the heart rate. In times of acute flare-up, you may need to have time in bed, but keep this as brief as possible and return to normal daily activity as quickly as you can.

Pacing or "Rhythm"

At Breathworks we've developed a systematic Mindfulness in Daily Life program that uses diary-keeping and analysis to help you become clearer about your tendencies and to enable you to live in a paced way. This means taking breaks *before* you get exhausted and using a timer to remind you to stop activities regularly.

❊ **BETTY**

I love pacing when it's going well. I don't always want to do it, and I find it frustrating, but it has transformed my life and opened possibilities that I didn't know I had, such as going out in the evening if I've rested. What I needed to understand was the concept of resting in advance of being tired. I'm used to pushing myself until I crash, so it was new for me to stop before I was exhausted. Then I move on to the next activity, feeling fresh rather than worn out.

In writing this book I've only worked at my computer for twenty minutes at a time because that's how long I can work before my pain increases. Then I lie down or gently putter around for fifteen minutes before returning to my computer for another twenty. In this way I can work for hours at a time, whereas if I were to do what I wanted without bringing mindfulness to my activities I'd work until the pain became unbearable, maybe an hour or two, and then be in a bad way for the rest of the day. I'm surprised at how much I can achieve with this steady and regular approach.

Do Something Enjoyable in Rest Periods

You're more likely to keep to pacing if you intersperse the activities you're pacing with an enjoyable, relaxing activity. For example, if you need to lie down regularly but find it hard to stop, you may find that reading a good book or magazine will help you keep to your pacing plans. If you don't enjoy your breaks you'll get frustrated and be more likely to keep going when you need to stop. Diane was a great fan of *The Sopranos*. She would do some housework for a timed period, then take a break and watch ten minutes of a *Sopranos* DVD before getting back to work.

In my own mindfulness rhythm of twenty minutes on the computer interspersed with fifteen minutes lying down, I've learned that I'm happiest when I read an undemanding novel with a good plot while I rest. Thrillers seem to fit the bill particularly well! I can easily reengage with my resting activity, and I don't feel as frustrated. Sometimes, of course, I want to hurl the timer across the room and ignore it when it's telling me to stop working—and sometimes I do! I can lose my awareness and push on for longer than twenty minutes, but I always pay the price in increased symptoms, so I've gradually accepted that pacing is really the only sustainable way to maintain a good quality of life when living with pain.

Jenny has back pain and has learned to bring mindfulness to her daily activities very well:

JENNY

I worked out that I could stand for about ten minutes without an increase in pain. If I'm doing dishes, I set the timer for ten minutes, and when it goes off I do something else, such as lying or sitting down for several minutes. Then I do the dishes for another ten minutes. It had never crossed my mind to do that. I had assumed that once you started doing dishes you carried on until you'd finished. It was revolutionary to think you could stop doing something many times, and then start it again.

I quickly learned I'd been drawing the wrong conclusion about the increases or decreases in my pain. I knew lying down often made it feel better, so I thought I should lie down for as much time as possible. I also noticed that going for a walk was sometimes beneficial, so I concluded that I should go for long walks. Neither strategy was helpful—I needed to learn that what I needed was frequent changes of activity. A fifteen-minute walk and a ten-minute lie-down were best, and any more lying down produced more pain.

This immediately gave me a sense of having a choice in dealing with pain rather than being a victim. I can't control all my external conditions, but I can be more conscious of the choices I make.

I've learned that to keep my pain within manageable limits, I need to lie down for five minutes every hour and a half. I can't sit at the computer for more than twenty minutes. I can walk for about an hour. I need to do various mindful movements every day, and I can hardly ever sit comfortably in a chair. I've also found, surprisingly, that I can sit in a moving car for three hours but on a train for one. The balance of my activities needs to be fine-tuned. For example, in my normal life I need more rest than most people, but on meditation retreats (which I regularly attend) I need to do more activity than everyone else.

THE THREE-MINUTE BREATHING SPACE

Another excellent way to bring mindfulness into everyday life is through a "three-minute breathing space." This is a pause in which you stop doing everything for three minutes. You sit quietly in a comfortable position, or if you prefer, you can stand, lie down, or adopt another posture of your choice. It's a great way to help you become more aware of what you're doing, how you're feeling, and so on, and you can usually find a way to fit a breathing space into your activities throughout the day at regular intervals. (A led version of the three-minute breathing space is available from soundstrue.com/burch.)

The first thing to do is to stop what you're doing and to be still, perhaps with your eyes closed (or half-closed). You can ask yourself, *How do I feel in my body at this moment?* and gradually allow yourself to become more aware of the various physical sensations in the body. Then allow yourself to experience the gentle movements of the body as you breathe. Where there's physical pain, take your attention to it with a kindly attitude, and let any muscles that have tightened around the pain soften on the in-breath and the out-breath. You can also become aware of how you're feeling emotionally and what sort of thoughts are passing through your mind.

If you remain aware of your breathing in this way, as well as of any sensations, feelings, and thoughts for at least three minutes, you'll probably find you become calmer and more centered and able to return to your activities with a fresh, more grounded perspective. This practice can help to interrupt a tendency to operate on autopilot, and you may find you regain the initiative in how you approach your activities.

You can use a timer to remind yourself to stop at regular intervals and to time the three minutes of the breathing space.

JANET

I find stopping very difficult. A three-minute meditation is useful in breaking up the frenzy that so quickly builds up in my daily life. Remembering to do it can be a problem, so I've learned to set a timer that goes off on the hour to remind myself that it's time to stop. I sit quietly for three minutes and bring my awareness back to my breath and my body, and I soon feel much calmer. It is such a simple and powerful way of bringing meditation and awareness into daily life.

MINDFULNESS OF EATING AND SLEEPING

When you're trying to live well with pain and illness it's easy to overlook obvious things such as eating well and establishing a regular sleeping routine. No amount of meditation makes up for three good meals a day and periods of restorative sleep, so it's important to pay attention to these areas if you want to establish a helpful mindfulness practice.

Pain and illness often lead people to lose their jobs, with a consequent loss of structure to the day. Health problems can also disrupt sleep, so you may find yourself staying up very late and then feeling continually exhausted and sleepy during the day. When you eventually drag yourself out of bed, the first thing you do is take medication, which makes you feel nauseous because you're taking it on an empty stomach.

Because you feel sick, you don't do your mindful stretches or meditate, and before you know it, you're in a downward slide toward poor diet, lack of exercise, and lack of motivation to meditate. You may even find that you never eat a proper nourishing meal.

If this is your situation, it can help to reestablish routines, making sure you eat breakfast before you take your pills and trying to sleep at night rather than during the day. It might take time to get yourself back on track, but you'll experience great rewards. Seek help from a professional if you need guidance on diet or sleep.

❋ JEREMY

Jeremy injured the nerves in his arm in a horrific motorcycle accident. He suffered intense nerve pain, and when he came to a Breathworks course he'd been unable to lie down to sleep for years. He was on heavy medication and had lost any sense of routine: watching TV during the day, staying up at night and feeling continually exhausted, snatching what sleep he could while sitting in a chair. He started practicing mindfulness and incorporated regular meals into his day, including breakfast, which he hadn't eaten for years. Slowly he established a routine that included regular meditation, and he started to feel much better. By attending to these basic daily routines he felt in charge of his life again for the first time since the accident.

AVOIDING HOLES IN THE SIDEWALK

If you bring mindfulness to all the elements of daily life in the ways I've described in this chapter, you will experience great benefits. This is where the awareness cultivated in formal meditation can flow into your behavior, radically improving your overall quality of life. As you make creative choices over and over again in all the little acts of everyday life, you can overcome unhelpful habits and learn new, helpful ones. It won't happen overnight, but steady practice will yield great results.

Autobiography in Five Short Chapters

Chapter One
I walk down the street.
There is a deep hole in the sidewalk.
I fall in.
I am lost . . . I am helpless.
It isn't my fault.
It takes forever to find a way out.

Chapter Two
I walk down the same street.
There is a deep hole in the sidewalk.
I pretend I don't see it.
I fall in again.
I can't believe I am in the same place.
But, it isn't my fault.
It still takes a long time to get out.

Chapter Three
I walk down the same street.
There is a deep hole in the sidewalk.
I see it is there.
I still fall in. It's a habit.
My eyes are open.
I know where I am.
It is my fault. I get out immediately.

Chapter Four
I walk down the same street.
There is a deep hole in the sidewalk.
I walk around it.

Chapter Five
I walk down another street.

PORTIA NELSON[1]

CHAPTER 18

Keep Going

Hour after hour, day
After day we try
To grasp the Ungraspable, pinpoint
The Unpredictable. Flowers
Wither when touched, ice
Suddenly cracks beneath our feet. Vainly
We try to track birdflight through the sky trace
Dumb fish through deep water, try
To anticipate the earned smile the soft
Reward, even
Try to grasp our own lives. But Life
Slips through our fingers
Like snow. Life
Cannot belong to us. We
Belong to Life. Life
Is King.
— SANGHARAKSHITA[1]

LIFE IS KING

In this book I've introduced a variety of ways in which you can use mindfulness to help you live well with pain and illness. Rather than just surviving, you can consciously choose life. This gives a profound sense of freedom as you take the initiative in both your inner and outer worlds, no longer a victim of your physical circumstances or your mental and emotional states.

But as Sangharakshita's poem says, ultimately *life is king,* and no matter how much you take responsibility for yourself and try to set up supportive routines and conditions, you cannot control all your circumstances. Things will happen that will throw you off course — for example, an illness that means you can't meditate or do any movement for a few days, and then when you get going again, you find you've lost fitness and momentum, and everything feels like a struggle. It might be a death in the family that plunges you into grief in which you lose your motivation to practice mindfulness, or you may have a fall or an accident that causes a flare-up of your symptoms, leaving you feeling more disabled than ever. These things happen; sometimes they seem to happen all at once, and it can be hard to remember the point of anything you've learned. I'll just say: don't give up altogether, and when you feel ready, *keep going!* Remember, it takes just one positive step in this moment to regain the initiative and move back toward life.

This has been one of the most important lessons for me in twenty years of practicing mindfulness while living with pain. I've had several severe setbacks in my condition due to overdoing it and also surgery. As a result, I've lost fitness, been too exhausted to meditate, and felt like a complete beginner when I eventually started to climb out of the pit into which I'd fallen. Each time I've slowly and steadily rehabilitated myself using the principles of awareness and pacing, and I've made it back to a stable level of functioning. Knowing I'm capable of rehabilitating myself from incapacity gives me greater confidence than the knowledge that I can practice when I am well.

Rachel had been off work with stress for several months before completing the Breathworks distance learning course. She shared the following tips in our web forum when she was ready to return to work.

RACHEL

In my occupational health interview this morning, I told the nurse how mindfulness had helped me to really feel what I was feeling, see how I was reacting, and manage my thinking during the time I'd been off work. I explained that my irritable bowel disease, stress, hypertension, and back pain had faded away for the most part. After I completed my practice, I felt an immediate change in my physical state.

Now that I'm getting busier, I can't meditate as much, and I find myself slipping back into old patterns of thinking and behaving, so this interview was a timely reminder of what exacerbated my pain, how it affected me, and what I need to do to maintain my well-being. My being is very well just now, and I want to keep it that way!

My suggestion is to take a moment to ask which aspects of mindfulness you find most helpful. Have you made them part of your daily routine? If you're feeling well, are you working on staying well? And if you're sliding back a little, what support do you need to get back on track?

These are good questions, and you'll need all the help you can get. Over the last seven years Harry has written down the strategies he's found useful so he has them to refer to when things are difficult.

HARRY

When my pain flares up I get out my file. It's like being my own personal adviser, and I think out a caring plan for when times are tough. I note anything that helps—meditation, exercises and relaxation techniques, tapes and CDs, books and inspiring quotes, and helpful tips from friends. I continually update my kit and modify it in the light of experience.

I hope you'll absorb the practices and ideas I've described in this book. Find out for yourself which ones are particularly useful for you and prepare your own "first-aid kit" to remind yourself of your intentions when your motivation wavers. You need to be prepared for setbacks —

an important part of mindfulness training is cultivating a deep and equanimous attitude to whatever happens and being willing to pick yourself up again and again, no matter how despondent you may feel. If you're well at the moment, then it's just as important, as Rachel says, to ask what you're doing to *stay* well.

THE JOURNEY CONTINUES

All the anecdotes in this book are from men and women just like you. They aren't special people — and neither am I. We're just trying the best we can to travel the path of awareness and become more fully alive and content. You can do this, too, and there will never be a better moment to practice than right now. Mindfulness practice never ends; it's a way of life, and I invite you to open yourself gently to the transformative power of breath awareness, mindful movement, and meditation. You'll learn an open secret, the miracle of mindfulness, that will help you to wake up to life just as it is and to live well, in all the moments, with as much dignity and inner peace as your circumstances allow. What are you waiting for?

Practice Schedule

Six key elements of the mindfulness program are introduced in this book:

1. Breath awareness
2. Mindful movement
3. Body scan
4. Mindfulness of breathing
5. Kindly awareness
6. Mindfulness in daily life

I recommend you include all these elements in your life in a balanced and consistent way. Inevitably you will like some better than others, but it's important to familiarize yourself thoroughly with them all. In Breathworks courses we teach these methods in an eight-week program. In using this book you should find your own pace, doing each of the practices for several weeks, ideally meditating at least six days out of seven each week. The main thing is to stick to them through the inevitable ups and downs.

SUGGESTED PROGRAM

Breath inquiry 3—whole body breathing: two weeks
Body scan: two weeks
Mindfulness of breathing: two weeks
Kindly awareness: two weeks

When you feel ready, I recommend you also start practicing mindful movement each day, if possible from week two onward. The mindfulness-in-daily-life module takes two weeks to establish and requires you to keep and analyze diaries. Incorporate this into your program when you feel ready, and then integrate pacing into your life to establish your own mindfulness rhythm.

This program is supported by an audio downloads, CDs, booklets, and a DVD. Please see soundstrue.com/burch and page 270 for details.

Pleasant and Unpleasant Events Diaries

I recommend you complete these diaries[1] as preparation for learning the kindly awareness meditation practice as outlined in chapter 15. Each day, be aware of one pleasant and one unpleasant event at the time it is happening. Use the questions to focus your awareness on the details of the experience. On page 232 is an example of how I filled in the diary. Photocopy the blank template (on page 233) and fill it in every day.

EXPERIENCE What was the experience?	AWARENESS Were you aware of the feelings *while* the event was happening?	SENSATION How did your body feel, in detail, during this experience?	EMOTION/ THOUGHTS What moods, feelings, and thoughts accompanied this event?	LEARNING Did you learn anything from this exercise?
SUNDAY **Pleasant** ☺ *Talking to friend in morning*	*Yes, gradually my mood changed during the conversation.*	*Tired and heavy to start with, but gradually more physically energized as my mood changed.*	*My friend's enthusiasm for life lifted my mood, my feelings became more positive, and my thoughts brightened and sharpened.*	*Fascinating how a good communication/ meeting with someone can change my experience: physically, mentally, and emotionally.*
SUNDAY **Unpleasant** ☹ *Tiredness and back pain mid-afternoon while on computer*	*Yes*	*Felt the tension of pushing the pain away – a sort of physical resistance.*	*Mood = low* *Feelings = frustration* *Thoughts = despair and self-pity*	*Glad that I've identified what happened. Know I can change physical, mental, and emotional experience by standing back from situation and having a rest.*
MONDAY **Pleasant** ☺ *Sitting in Jacuzzi!*	*Yes*	*Soothed, though achy; calmed.*	*A sense of real pleasure. Happy feelings, moods, thoughts.*	*I must prioritize this activity and remember how beneficial it is!*
MONDAY **Unpleasant** ☹ *A difficult communication*	*Yes*	*Very tight and I was angry and tense. Felt hot, agitated, extreme back pain.*	*Struggled not to react aggressively. Felt under intense strain mentally. Thoughts of not being able to cope.*	*It is so clear how difficult emotional states can aggravate my perception of pain. Proves the importance of meditation and awareness practices to help build emotional stability.*

EXPERIENCE What was the experience?	AWARENESS Were you aware of the feelings *while* the event was happening?	SENSATION How did your body feel, in detail, during this experience?	EMOTION/ THOUGHTS What moods, feelings, and thoughts accompanied this event?	LEARNING Did you learn anything from this exercise?
Pleasant ☺				
Unpleasant ☹				
Pleasant ☺				
Unpleasant ☹				

Finding Out More

RESOURCES

Mindfulness and meditation practice are easier to maintain if you have aids that help you to be as comfortable as possible. Below is a list of items that may help.

Lying-Down Postures

- You can buy meditation mats or yoga mats for comfort.
- A yoga bolster can help to ease pressure on the spine, if placed under the knees.
- An eye pillow may help the eyes to relax.

If You Kneel to Meditate

You can use any of the following:

- Meditation cushions (sometimes called a *zafu*).
- A meditation stool (a small wooden stool to slide your knees underneath).
- Yoga blocks (I find two blocks measuring 12 x 8 x 2 inches is a good size.)
- A rubber stability cushion inflated to the correct height and placed on top of the yoga blocks is an excellent way to take the strain off the spine and sacrum. These are marketed as "stability cushions," "wobble cushions," "balance cushions," or "airdisks."

If You Sit on a Chair to Meditate

Use any ordinary straight-backed chair. If you can't comfortably rest your feet flat on the floor, it can help to place a firm cushion beneath your feet (e.g., a meditation cushion/zafu), and a stability cushion may relieve pressure beneath your sacrum and sitting bones.

Mindful Movement

Use a yoga mat, exercise mat, folded blanket, or meditation mat for comfort. If you have trouble reaching around the legs during the relevant postures, use a belt, yoga strap, or scarf to help you.

Mindfulness in Daily Life and Timing Meditations

It helps to invest in a timer to assist you with your pacing/mindfulness rhythm. Any digital countdown timer will do, but ideally find a product that has at least two rotating cycles so you can alternate activity and rest cycles, e.g., fifteen minutes working and five minutes lying down on a continuous rotating cycle. Timex Ironman watches have this feature (called a "countdown interval timer"). At Breathworks we sell versions that vibrate (rather than with an audible alarm), which are good for use in public situations and timing meditations.

GOING FURTHER WITH MEDITATION

Breathworks Courses

A Breathworks course is an ideal introduction to the material in this book, with the support and encouragement of a tutor and other participants. If you can't access a course locally, you can follow the course from anywhere in the world by distance learning with weekly telephone and/ or e-mail support. For further details, visit the Breathworks website at breathworks-mindfulness.co.uk.

Online Meditation Instruction and Resources

1. Soundstrue.com/guide/meditation
2. Wildmind.org offers a comprehensive program of online meditation instruction and support. They also stock a wide range of CDs of led practices.
3. Meditationforeveryone.com: The Clear Vision Trust has produced an introductory DVD *Meditation for Everyone*.
4. Dharma.org (Insight Meditation Society)
5. Mindfulnessprograms.com

Retreats

A residential retreat is an ideal way to consolidate your learning and practice in supportive and beautiful conditions. I regularly run retreats in the United Kingdom at Taraloka Women's Buddhist Retreat Center (taraloka.org.uk) as well as at other venues in Great Britain and internationally. Contact the Breathworks office for my schedule (info@breathworks.co.uk) and other Breathworks-related retreats.

From my personal knowledge and experience I can recommend activities run by the Friends of the Western Buddhist Order (FWBO). Information on retreat centers associated with this movement is available at goingonretreat.com. For details of activities and classes in other countries, see fwbo.org. Some retreats are based on Buddhist teachings and practices while others focus on yoga, tai chi, hill walking, creative expression, and so on.

Here are some other recommended centers that teach mindfulness meditation:

1. Insight Meditation Society, Barre, Massachusetts, dharma.org
2. Spirit Rock, Woodacre, California, spiritrock.org
3. Menla Mountain Retreat and Conference Center, Phoenicia, New York, menla.org

4. Shambhala Mountain Center, Red Feather Lakes, Colorado, shambhalamountain.org
5. Blue Cliff Monastery, Pine Bush, New York, bluecliffmonastery.org

Mindfulness and Health

Some centers specialize in mindfulness-based stress reduction (MBSR) and mindfulness-based cognitive therapy (MBCT).

1. Center for Mindfulness, University of Massachusetts Medical School, Worcester, Massachusetts.
    E-mail: mindfulness@umassmed.edu
    Website: umassmed.edu/cfm
2. USCD (University of California, San Diego) Center for Mindfulness, La Jolla, California. mindfulness.ucsd.edu
3. For more information on the dialogue between modern science and Buddhism, please visit the Mind and Life Institute at mindandlife.org.

Notes

Foreword

1. Jon Kabat-Zinn and others, "Four Year Follow-Up of a Meditation-Based Program for the Self-Regulation of Chronic Pain: Treatment Outcomes and Compliance," *Clinical Journal of Pain 2* (1986): 159–173.
2. Lance McCracken, Jeremy Gauntlet-Gilbert, and Kevin Vowles, "The Role of Mindfulness in a Contextual Cognitive-Behavioural Analysis of Chronic Pain-Related Suffering and Disability," *Pain* (IASP) 131 (September 2007): 63–69.

Introduction

1. Stephen Levine and Ondrea Levine, *Who Dies?* (New York: Anchor, 1989).

Chapter 1

1. Harald Breivik and others, "Survey of Chronic Pain in Europe: Prevalence, Impact on Daily Life, and Treatment," *European Journal of Pain* 10 (2006): 287–333. This was a large-scale, computer-assisted, telephone-interview study undertaken to explore the prevalence, severity, treatment, and impact of chronic pain in fifteen European countries and Israel.
2. "Pain in America: A Research Report," Gallup Organization for Merck & Co, Inc., Ogilvy Public Relations, 2000.
3. See appendix 3, page 238, for more information on the Center for Mindfulness and other mindfulness-based approaches.
4. See chapter 4 for more on this.

Chapter 2

1. "Classification of Chronic Pain," *Pain* (IASP) Suppl. (1986): 53.
2. Quoted in Patrick Wall, *Pain: The Science of Suffering* (London: Weidenfeld & Nicolson, 1999), 29.
3. Michael Bond and Karen Simpson, *Pain: Its Nature and Treatment* (Edinburgh: Elsevier, 2006), 4.
4. Frances Cole and others, *Overcoming Chronic Pain* (London: Constable & Robinson, 2005), 37. Bond and Simpson (*Pain*, 16) offer an alternative definition from the International Association for the Study of Pain as acute pain (lasting less than one month), subacute pain (one to six months), and chronic pain (six months or more).
5. See Patrick Wall for one such definition.
6. M. C. Jensen, "Magnetic Resonance Imaging of the Lumbar Spine in People without Back Pain," *New England Journal of Medicine* 331, no. 2 (July 1994): 69–73.
7. Wilbert Fordyce and others, "Pain Measurement and Pain Behavior," *Pain* 18 (1984): 53–69; A. Gamsa, "The Role of Psychological Factors in Chronic Pain I: A Half Century of Study," *Pain* 57, no. 1 (April 1994): 5–15.
8. Patrick Wall, *Pain*, 78.
9. Patrick Wall and Ronald Melzack, *The Challenge of Pain* (New York: Penguin, 1982), 98.
10. Patrick Wall, *Pain*, 31.

Chapter 3

1. See, for example, the work of the Mind and Life Institute: mindandlife.org.
2. Samyutta Nikaya 36. 6: Sallatha Sutta, "The Arrow."
3. Ibid.
4. Ibid.

5. Ibid.
6. Ibid.
7. Ibid.

Chapter 4

1. Amy Schmidt, *Dipa Ma: The Life and Legacy of a Buddhist Master* (New York: Blue Bridge, 2005), 42.
2. Analayo, "The Satipatthana Sutta," *Satipatthana: The Direct Path to Realisation* (Cambridge, UK: Windhorse Publications, 2003), 3–13.
3. Jon Kabat-Zinn, *Wherever You Go, There You Are: Mindfulness Meditation in Everyday Life* (London: Piatkus, 2004), 4.
4. Mark Williams and others, *The Mindful Way Through Depression: Freeing Yourself from Chronic Unhappiness* (New York: Guildford Press, 2007), 48.
5. Ibid, 5.
6. Pierre Hadot, *Philosophy as a Way of Life* (Hoboken, NJ: Wiley-Blackwell, 1995), 84–5.
7. B. Alan Wallace and Shauna L. Shapiro, "Mental Balance and Well-being: Building Bridges between Buddhism and Western Science," *American Psychologist* 61, no. 7 (October 2006): 690–701.
8. Analayo, *Satipatthana*, 58.
9. Analayo, *Satipatthana*, 46–7, discusses the connection between the word *sati* and memory.
10. Sangharakshita, *Living with Awareness* (Cambridge, UK: Windhorse Publications, 2003), 21.
11. This is described within *satipatthana* meditation as the quality of *sampajanna*, variously translated as "mindfulness of purpose," "clear comprehension," or "clearly knowing." See Analayo *Satipatthana*, 39, and Sangharakshita *Living with Awareness*, 13.

12. Sangharakshita, *Living with Awareness*, 23. Simple awareness (*sati*) and comprehension of purpose or clearly knowing (*sampajanna*) often appear as a compound term in the Buddhist tradition: *satisampajanna*. The two words are so close in meaning as to be virtually interchangeable, and yet there is no precise word in English that does justice to the qualities they evoke. Awareness and knowledge are both essential to leading a creative life.

13. Sangharakshita, *Living with Awareness*, 140.

14. Analayo, *Satipatthana*, 54.

15. Jon Kabat-Zinn, "Mindfulness-Based Interventions in Context: Past, Present, and Future," *Clinical Psychology: Science and Practice* 10 (2003): 145.

16. Bhikkuni Kusuma, *A Mental Therapy: The Development of the Four Foundations of Mindfulness, or Sati Satipatthana, in Theravada Buddhist Meditation (Vipassana)* (Taiwan: The Corporate Body of the Buddha Educational Foundation), 5.

17. See Analayo, *Satipatthana*, 29–30.

18. The fourth dimension of mindfulness is *dhammas*. The interpretation I find most useful is that it provides a perspective based on truth from which you can regard your experience. See Analayo, *Satipatthana*, 183.

19. From the *Vajracchedika-prajnaparamita*, "The Diamond Sutra," xxxii. This translation is by Dr. Kenneth Saunders, reproduced in *The Diamond Sutra & The Sutra of Hui-neng*, trans. A. F. Price and Wong Mou-lam (Boston: Shambhala Publications, 1969), 530.

20. This is another way of looking at *dhammas*. The principle of conditionality — that all things arise and fall in dependence on causes and conditions — means you can gradually guide your life in the direction of the good.

21. Jeffrey Hopkins, *Cultivating Compassion* (New York: Broadway Books, 2001), 32.

22. Rainer Maria Rilke, "The Dove That Ventured Outside," in *Ahead of All Parting: The Selected Poetry and Prose of Rainer Maria Rilke,* trans. Stephen Mitchell (New York: Modern Library, 1995).
23. This image appears in a Buddhist scripture called *The Avatamsaka Sutra.* See also Francis H. Cook, *Hua-Yen Buddhism: The Jewel Net of Indra* (Pennsylvania State University, 1977).

Chapter 5

1. Rumi, "Quietness," in *Rumi: Selected Poems,* trans. Coleman Barks (London: Penguin, 1995), 22.
2. Charlotte Joko Beck, *Everyday Zen* (London: Thorsons, 1989), 47.
3. Jon Kabat-Zinn, *Full Catastrophe Living* (New York: Delta, 2005), 264.

Chapter 6

1. Rainer Maria Rilke, *Ahead of All the Parting: The Selected Poetry and Prose of Rainer Maria Rilke,* trans. Stephen Mitchell (New York: Modern Library, 1995), 91.
2. Jon Kabat-Zinn, *Wherever You Go,* 162–3.
3. Jon Kabat-Zinn, *Wherever You Go,* 168.
4. Stephen Levine, *Healing into Life and Death* (New York: Anchor Books, 1989).
5. She lists denial, anger, bargaining, depression, and acceptance. Elisabeth Kübler-Ross, *On Death and Dying* (New York: Scribner, 1997).
6. Matthew Sandford, *Waking: A Memoir of Trauma and Transcendence* (Emmaus, PA: Rodale Publications, 2006), 127–8.
7. Ibid, 128.
8. Ibid, 127.
9. Ibid, 193, 194, 199.

10. Ibid, 198.
11. Ibid, 182.
12. Mary Oliver, "Wild Geese" in *Dream Work* (New York: Grove/ Atlantic, Inc., 1986).

Chapter 7

1. Rumi, "The Turn: Dance in Your Blood," in *The Essential Rumi* (Edison, NJ: Castle, 1998), 267.
2. James Joyce, *Dubliners* (New York: Penguin Modern Classics, 2000).
3. Eric Partridge, *A Short Etymological Dictionary of Modern English* (Routledge and Kegan Paul, 1963). "Rehabilitation" comes from Latin *habere*, meaning "to hold, hence to occupy, hence to have." It is the common root of words such as *habitation, habit, rehabilitate.*
4. Gavin Burt, "It's Your Move," *Talkback Magazine* (Autumn 2007), 15.
5. See also Donna Farhi, *The Breathing Book* (New York: Henry Holt, 1996).
6. For more on common ways of inhibiting the breath, see Donna Farhi, *The Breathing Book*, 98.
7. Donna Farhi, *The Breathing Book*, 98.
8. Mu Soeng, *Trust in Mind,* trans. Stanley Lombardo (Boston: Wisdom Publications, 2004), 142.
9. For more on the qualities of optimal breathing, see Donna Farhi, *The Breathing Book*, 45–6.

Chapter 8

1. Rumi, *Rumi: Selected Poems,* trans. Coleman Barks (London: Penguin, 1995), 174.
2. Ruth Dickstein and Judith E. Deutsch, "Motor Imagery in Physical Therapist Practice," *Physical Therapy* 87, no. 7 (July 2007): 942–53.

Chapter 9

1. Ryokan, *Great Fool* (Honolulu: University of Hawai'i Press, 1996), 153.
2. Ruth A. Baer, "Mindfulness Training as a Clinical Intervention: A Conceptual and Empirical Review," *Clinical Psychology: Science and Practice* 10, no. 2 (2003): 125–43.
3. .For more details see the research page on Breathworks website at breathworks-mindfulness.co.uk.
4. Paul Grossman and others, "Mindfulness-Based Stress Reduction and Health Benefits: A Meta-Analysis," *Journal of Psychosomatic Research* 57, no. 1 (2004): 35–43.
5. K. Proulx, "Integrating Mindfulness-Based Stress Reduction," *Holistic Nursing Practice* 17, no. 4 (2003): 201–8.
6. "The Effectiveness of Meditation Techniques to Reduce Blood Pressure Levels: A Meta-Analysis," *Dissertation Abstracts International* 47, no. 11–B (1987): 4639.
7. Richard Davidson and others, "Alterations in Brain and Immune Function Produced by Mindfulness Meditation," *Psychosomatic Medicine* 65, no. 4 (2003): 564–70.
8. The National Institutes of Health, "Alternative Medicine: Expanding Medical Horizons," *A Report to the National Institutes of Health on Alternative Medical Systems and Practices in the United States,* NIH Publication no. 94-066 (1994).
9. These are translations of terms from the Buddhist tradition of meditation teaching, especially associated with the sixth-century Buddhist meditation master Chih-i. "Stopping" translates *samatha,* and "seeing" translates *vipassana.*
10. Pema Chödrön, *Good Medicine.* CD. Sounds True, 1999.

Chapter 10

1. David Whyte, *Where Many Rivers Meet* (Langley, Washington: Many Rivers Press, 1990), 2.

2. Larry Rosenberg, *Breath by Breath* (Boston: Shambhala Publications, 1998), 33.
3. Adapted from Kosho Uchiyama's *Opening the Hand of Thought* (Boston: Wisdom Publications, 2005), 54.
4. Monty Roberts, *The Man Who Listens to Horses* (New York: Random House, 1997).
5. Sayadaw U. Tejanaya, "The Wise Investigator," *Tricycle: The Buddhist Review* (Winter 2001): 44.
6. Lecture to conference on mindfulness-based stress reduction, University of Wales, Bangor, 2001.
7. Shunryu Suzuki, *Zen Mind, Beginner's Mind*, trans. John Stevens (New York: Weatherhill, 1973), epigraph.

Chapter 11

1. Rumi, *Hidden Music*, trans. Maryam Mafi and Azima Melita Kolin (London: Thorsons, 2001), 90.

Chapter 13

1. Rainer Maria Rilke, *Rilke's Book of Hours: Love Poems to God*, trans. Anita Barrows and Joanna Macy (New York: Riverhead, 1996), 171.
2. Suzuki, *Zen Mind*, 46.
3. William Hart, *Vipassana Meditation* (New York: Harper Collins, 1987), 91.

Chapter 14

1. Analayo, *Satipatthana*, 267.

Chapter 15

1. *Sutta Nipata* 1. 8: The Karaniya Metta Sutta, "Loving Kindness."
2. *Collins English Dictionary* (Glasgow, 1979).
3. Lecture to conference on mindfulness-based approaches, University of Wales, Bangor, 2006.

Chapter 16

1. Zinden Segal, Mark Williams, and John Teasdale, *Mindfulness-Based Cognitive Therapy for Depression: A New Approach for Preventing Relapse* (New York: Guildford Press, 2002), 244.

2. Spencer Smith and Steven Hayes, *Get Out of Your Mind and Into Your Life* (Oakland, CA: New Harbinger Publications, 2005), 66. The phrase "looking at thoughts rather than from them" also comes from this book.

3. The term *emotional charge* is used by Jon Kabat-Zinn, *Wherever You Go*, 68.

4. Spencer Smith and Steven Hayes, *Get Out of Your Mind*, 32 and 66.

5. Thanks to Segal, Williams, and Teasdale, *Mindfulness-Based Cognitive Therapy*, 250, for this and the two following images of "sky and clouds" and "leaves on a stream."

6. These similes were first used by the Buddha. Bhikkhu Bodhi, *The Connected Discourses of the Buddha: A Translation of the Samyutta Nikaya* (Boston: Wisdom Publications, 2000), 1611–13.

7. Jeffrey Hopkins, *Cultivating Compassion*, 13.

Chapter 17

1. Portia Nelson, *There's a Hole in My Sidewalk* (Hillsboro, OR: Beyond Words Publishing, 1993).

Chapter 18

1. Sangharakshita, *Complete Poems* (Cambridge, UK: Windhorse Publications, 1995), 285.

Appendix 2

1. Adapted from Jon Kabat-Zinn, *Full Catastrophe Living* (London: Piatkus, 2005), 446–47.

Further Reading

Meditation and Mindfulness

Analayo. *Satipatthana: The Direct Path to Realisation,* Cambridge, UK: Windhorse Publications, 2003.

Bodhipaksa. *Wildmind: A Step-by-step Guide to Meditation,* Cambridge, UK: Windhorse Publications, 2007.

Hart, W. *Vipassana Meditation: The Art of Living As Taught by S. N. Goenka,* New York: HarperCollins, 1987.

Kabat-Zinn, J. *Wherever You Go, There You Are: Mindfulness Meditation in Everyday Life,* New York: Hyperion, 2005.

Kamalashila. *Meditation: Buddhist Way of Tranquillity and Insight,* Cambridge, UK: Windhorse Publications, 2003.

Paramananda. *Change Your Mind,* Cambridge, UK: Windhorse Publications, 1996.

Rosenberg, L. *Breath by Breath,* London: Thorsons, 1998.

Sangharakshita. *Living with Awareness,* Cambridge, UK: Windhorse Publications, 2003.

Buddhism

Beck, C. J. *Everyday Zen,* London: Thorsons, 1989.

———. *Nothing Special: Living Zen,* San Francisco: HarperSanFrancisco, 1995.

Bodhi, Bhikkhu. *In the Buddha's Words: An Anthology of Discourses from the Pali Canon,* Boston: Wisdom Publications, 2005.

Hopkins, J. *Cultivating Compassion,* New York: Broadway Books, 2001.

Kulananda. *Principles of Buddhism,* Cambridge, UK: Windhorse Publications, 2006.

Nanamoli, Bhikkhu. *The Life of the Buddha According to the Pali Canon*, Onalaska, Washington: Pariyatti Publishing, 2001.

Saltzburg, S. *A Heart as Wide as the World*, Boston: Shambhala Publications, 1997.

Sangharakshita. *A Guide to the Buddhist Path*, Cambridge, UK: Windhorse Publications, 2006.

_____. *The Three Jewels: The Central Ideals of Buddhism*, Cambridge, UK: Windhorse Publications, 1998.

_____. *What Is the Dharma? The Essential Teachings of the Buddha*, Cambridge, UK: Windhorse Publications, 2007.

_____. *What Is the Sangha? The Nature of Spiritual Community*, Cambridge, UK: Windhorse Publications, 2001.

_____. *Who Is the Buddha?* Cambridge, UK: Windhorse Publications, 2002.

Schmidt, A. *Dipa Ma: The Life and Legacy of a Buddhist Master*, New York: Blue Bridge, 2005.

Sogyal Rinpoche. *The Tibetan Book of Living and Dying: A Spiritual Classic from One of the Foremost Interpreters of Tibetan Buddhism to the West*, New York: Random House, 2002.

Suzuki, S. *Zen Mind, Beginner's Mind*, Boston: Shambhala, 2006.

Thich Nhat Hanh. *The Miracle of Mindfulness*, Boston: Beacon Press, 1999.

Vajragupta. *Buddhism: Tools for Living Your Life*, Cambridge, UK: Windhorse Publications, 2007.

Health

Bertherat, T. and C. Bernstein. *The Body Has Its Reasons*, Rochester, VT: Healing Arts Press, 1989.

Farhi, D. *The Breathing Book*, New York: Henry Holt & Company, 1996.

Kabat-Zinn, J. *Coming to Our Senses*, New York: Hyperion, 2006.

_____. *Full Catastrophe Living*, New York: Delta, 1990.

Klein, A. *Chronic Pain: The Complete Guide to Relief*, London: Carroll & Graf Publishing, 2001.

Kübler-Ross E., *On Death and Dying,* New York: Simon and Schuster, 1997.

Levine, S. and Levine, O. *Who Dies?* New York: Anchor, 1989.

Levine, S. *Healing into Life and Death,* New York: Anchor, 1989.

Santorelli, S. *Heal Thy Self: Lessons on Mindfulness in Medicine,* New York: Three Rivers Press, 2000.

Segal, Z., M. Williams, and J. Teasdale, *Mindfulness-Based Cognitive Therapy for Depression: A New Approach for Preventing Relapse,* New York: Guildford Press, 2002.

Smith, S. and S. Hayes, *Get Out of Your Mind and Into Your Life: The New Acceptance and Commitment Therapy,* New Harbinger Publications, 2005.

Williams, M., Z. Segal, J. Teasdale, and J. Kabat-Zinn, *The Mindful Way Through Depression: Freeing Yourself From Chronic Unhappiness,* New York: Guildford Press, 2007.

Accounts of Managing Health Difficulties with Awareness or Meditation

Bedard, J. *Lotus in the Fire: The Healing Power of Zen,* Boston: Shambhala Publications, 1999.

Boucher, S. *Hidden Spring: A Buddhist Woman Confronts Cancer,* Boston: Wisdom Publications, 2000.

Cohen, D. *Turning Suffering Inside Out: A Zen Approach to Living with Physical and Emotional Pain,* Boston: Shambhala Publications, 2003.

Rosenbaum, E. *Here for Now: Living Well with Cancer Through Mindfulness,* Hardwick, MA: Satya House Publications, 2007.

Sadler, J. *Pain Relief without Drugs,* Rochester, VT: Healing Arts Press, 2007.

Sandford, M., *Waking: A Memoir of Trauma and Transcendence,* Emmaus, PA: Rodale Publications, 2006.

Shone N. *Coping Successfully with Pain,* London: Sheldon Press, 1995.

Pain

Bond, M. and K. Simpson. *Pain: Its Nature and Treatment,* Edinburgh: Elsevier, 2006.

Cole, F., H. Macdonald, C. Carus, and H. Howden-Leach. *Overcoming Chronic Pain,* London: Constable & Robinson, 2005.

Nicholas, M., A. Molloy, L. Tonkin, and L. Beeston. *Manage Your Pain,* London: Souvenir Press, 2003.

Padfield, D. *Perceptions of Pain,* Stockport, UK: Dewi Lewis Publications, 2003.

Wall, P. and R. Melzack. *The Challenge of Pain,* New York: Penguin Books, 1982.

Wall, P. *Pain: The Science of Suffering,* London: Weidenfeld & Nicolson, 1999.

Poetry

Oliver, M. *New and Selected Poems,* Boston: Beacon Press, 1992.

Rilke, R. M. *Ahead of All Parting: The Selected Poetry and Prose of Rainer Maria Rilke.* Translated by Stephen Mitchell. New York: Modern Library, 1995.

———. *Rilke's Book of Hours: Love Poems to God.* Translated by A. Barrows and J. Macy. New York: Riverhead, 2005.

Rumi. *The Essential Rumi.* Translated by Coleman Barks. Edison, NJ: Castle, 1998.

———. *Hidden Music.* Translated by M. Mafi and A. M. Kolin. London: Thorsons, 2001.

———. *Rumi: Selected Poems.* Translated by Coleman Barks. London: Penguin, 1995.

Ryokan. *Great Fool: Zen Master Ryokan — Poems, Letters, and Other Writings.* Translated by P. Haskel and R. Abe. Honolulu: University of Hawai'i Press, 1996.

———. *One Robe, One Bowl.* Translated by John Stevens. New York: Weatherhill Press, 1997.

Sangharakshita. *Complete Poems,* Cambridge, UK: Windhorse Publications, 1995.

Whyte, D. *Where Many Rivers Meet,* Langley, WA: Many Rivers Press, 1990.

Other

Hadot, P. *Philosophy as a Way of Life,* Hoboken, NJ: Wiley-Blackwell, 1995.

Nelson, P. *There's a Hole in My Sidewalk,* Hillsboro, OR: Beyond Words Publishing, 1994.

Roberts, M. *The Man Who Listens to Horses,* New York: Random House, 1997.

Index

About the Author

Originally from New Zealand, Vidyamala Burch sustained a spinal injury when she was sixteen, leaving her with persistent pain and partial paraplegia. Twenty years ago she started exploring mindfulness and meditation techniques to manage her own condition, which led her to move to the United Kingdom, where she was based at a residential retreat center for five years and was ordained into the Western Buddhist Order.

In 2001 she felt ready to offer the fruits of her long personal experience of using meditation and mindfulness to live well with pain, and ran a pilot scheme in Manchester, England, for others wanting to learn the methods she had developed. The success of this led to her founding the Breathworks organization in 2004 with two close colleagues, Sona Fricker and Gary Hennessey (Ratnaguna). Breathworks is dedicated to offering mindfulness-based approaches for the benefit of anyone who experiences suffering, and it is now established in thirteen countries. Vidyamala is involved in training others to deliver the program, as well as offering courses herself in Manchester.

As a member of the Western Buddhist Order, Vidyamala also leads intensive meditation retreats regularly. Visit her website at breathworks-mindfulness.co.uk.

About Sounds True

Sounds True was founded in 1985 with a clear vision: to disseminate spiritual wisdom. Located in Boulder, Colorado, Sounds True publishes teaching programs that are designed to educate, uplift, and inspire. We work with many of the leading spiritual teachers, thinkers, healers, and visionary artists of our time.

To receive a free catalog of tools and teachings for personal and spiritual transformation, please visit soundstrue.com, call toll free at 800-333-9185, or write to us at the address below.

SOUNDS TRUE
PO Box 8010 / Boulder, CO 80306